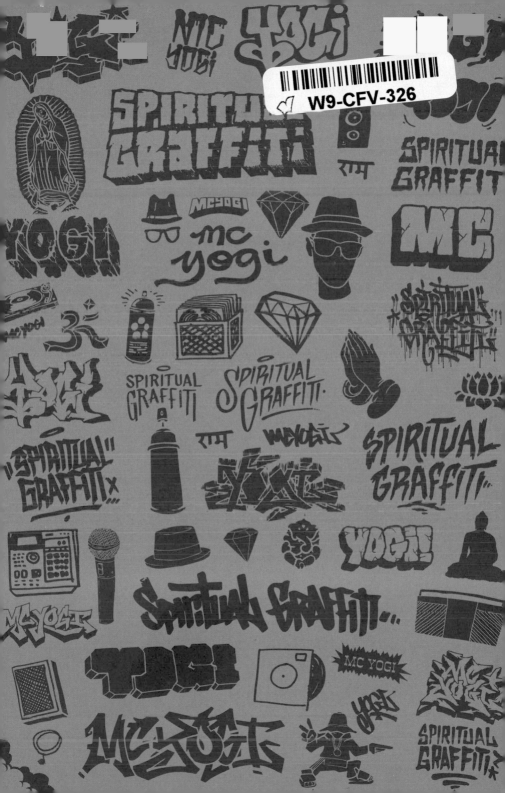

ADVANCE PRAISE FOR SPIRITUAL GRAFFITI

"Behind the music and off the mat—MC YOGI's story of grit and graffiti reminds us that yoga meets us wherever we are and introduces us to who we are."

—**Jason Mraz, multi-platinum and Grammy-winning musician**

"Let MC's journey be a reminder to inspire you to follow your own spiritual heart."

—**Jack Kornfield, founder of Spirit Rock Center**

"MC YOGI's hot, hip, and holy book, *Spiritual Graffiti,* tells the story of a modern-day prophet whose soul journey from darkness to light illustrates that with great love all is possible."

—**Sharon Gannon, founder of Jivamukti Yoga**

"The first time I set my eyes on MC YOGI, I said, 'There is a man who can help change the world!' He speaks the language, sings the songs, and carries the rhythm of the generations who are ready to bring this world into the age of peace."

—**Gurmukh, founder of Golden Bridge Yoga**

"MC YOGI is a revolutionary drawing on the power of music, yoga, art, and activism in a new genre of conscious hip-hop. *Spiritual Graffiti* is a vulnerable and inspiring message that is a gift to all."

—**Shiva Rea, founder Samdura Global School of Living Yoga**

"MC YOGI's journey of hard times, confusion, and discouragement has garnered him a potent voice for balance, clarity, and hope."

—**DJ Drez, music producer and international DJ**

"I read this book in one sitting. It was a great read. So good to see how MC YOGI's light found a way to triumph over such great adversity."

—**Krishna Das, Grammy-nominated musician**

"*Spiritual Graffiti* is a journey of awakening and a call to revolution! MC YOGI is one of my favorite Comrades in the fight against greed, hatred, and delusion."

—**Noah Levine, author of *Dharma Punx* and *Refuge Recovery***

"I can't wait to hand MC YOGI's *Spiritual Graffiti* to my students. They will recognize themselves in his stories of a chaotic childhood and find hope in his quest for big dreams and big love, even as he travels his own road home."

—**Jessica Lahey, *New York Times* bestselling author of *The Gift of Failure***

"*Spiritual Graffiti* highlights the inexhaustible powers of yoga to change lives and lay down a path that can uplift, even in the darkest hours of our life. Inspiring, heartwarming, and deeply encouraging: a must-read."

—**Janet Stone, international yoga teacher and founder of Janet Stone Yoga**

"Through MC YOGI's honest storytelling we see and then believe his assertion that with great love, anything is possible."

—**Kathryn Budig, yoga teacher, author, and co-host of espnW's podcast *Free Cookies***

"When MC YOGI raps, people listen. How lucky we are now to get the story behind the killer beats. The writing is on the wall: *Spiritual Graffiti* is one for the ages!"

—**Leza Lowitz, author of *Yoga Poems*: *Lines to Unfold By* and *Here Comes the Sun***

"The path MC YOGI has forged is unforgettable, and his book is needed. May all of us learn to rise up in our own way reading his wise and true understandings."

—**Elena Brower, author of *Practice You* and *Art of Attention***

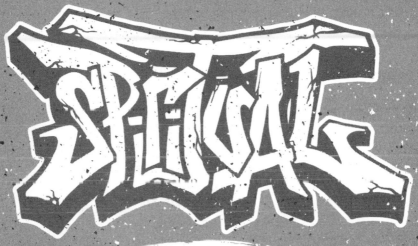

SPIRITUAL

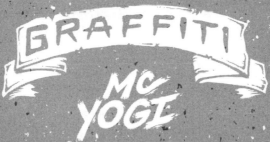

GRAFFITI

MC YOGI

HarperOne
An Imprint of HarperCollinsPublishers

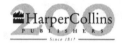

SPIRITUAL GRAFFITI. Copyright © 2017 by MC YOGI. All rights reserved. Printed in the United States of America. No part of this book may be used or reproduced in any manner whatsoever without written permission except in the case of brief quotations embodied in critical articles and reviews. For information, address HarperCollins Publishers, 195 Broadway, New York, NY 10007.

HarperCollins books may be purchased for educational, business, or sales promotional use. For information, please email the Special Markets Department at SPsales@harpercollins.com.

FIRST EDITION

Designed by Janet M. Evans-Scanlon

Illustrations by MC YOGI

Library of Congress Cataloging-in-Publication Data is available upon request.

ISBN 978-0-06-257253-0

17 18 19 20 21 LSC 10 9 8 7 6 5 4 3 2 1

DEDICATED TO MY
WIFE AND BEST
FRIEND

"AMANDA"

THANK YOU FOR
WALKING ME HOME

TABLE OF

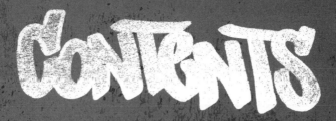

CONTENTS

"WHEN YOU ARE INSPIRED BY SOME GREAT PURPOSE, SOME EXTRAORDINARY PROJECT, ALL YOUR THOUGHTS BREAK THEIR BONDS: YOUR MIND TRANSCENDS LIMITATIONS, YOUR CONSCIOUSNESS EXPANDS IN EVERY DIRECTION, AND YOU FIND YOURSELF IN A NEW, GREAT AND WONDERFUL WORLD. DORMANT FORCES, FACULTIES AND TALENTS BECOME ALIVE, AND YOU DISCOVER YOURSELF TO BE A GREATER PERSON BY FAR THAN YOU EVER DREAMED YOURSELF TO BE."

- PATANJALI

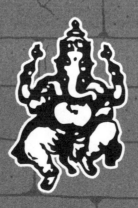

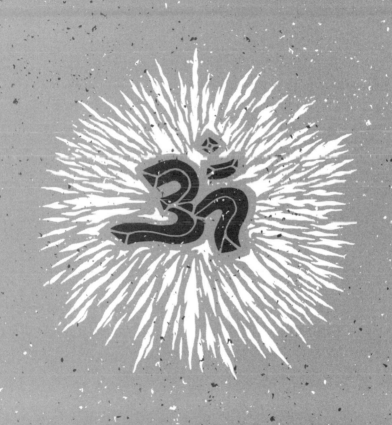

1

OM

THIS IS IT, I THOUGHT. IT WAS BY FAR THE LARGEST audience I'd ever performed to. I stood on the front edge of the stage, gazing out at the massive crowd. Looking out, I could see ten thousand pairs of eyes staring back at me. I marveled at all the twists and turns that my life had taken, the wild and unexpected journey that had led me to this moment. My entire being swelled with energy as adrenaline pumped through my bloodstream. I felt the anticipation of the crowd. I prayed I would remember all my lyrics and be able to hit all my cues. I took a deep breath in.

"ARE YOU REEEEAAAADDDDDYYYY?" My voice echoed through the sound system as I called out to the crowd. The entire festival hollered back with applause and cheers of excitement. "Let's count it off together!" I shouted. "TEN." The crowd joined in. "NINE." There was a rush as everyone pushed closer toward the stage.

"EIGHT. . . . Everybody get low," I called out. "SEVEN." The whole audience crouched down toward the earth. "SIX." I could see security flanking either side of the stage at full attention. "FIVE." I joined the crowd and knelt onstage. "FOUR. . . . Get ready!" I yelled. "THREE." I could see the excitement building in everybody's eyes. "TWO." I looked at my DJ, his hand hovering over the record, ready to drop the beat. "ONNNNEEE!!"

BOOM! As the beat dropped, the entire crowd leapt up, releasing handfuls of colored dust. It was a psychedelic explosion of pure love. Huge plumes of bright blue, magenta pink, and neon green exploded in the air, streaking across the sky. For a moment I couldn't see anything except an endless haze of rainbow colors and dust. And then, as the clouds of color washed over the crowd, I saw one of the most beautiful things I've ever witnessed in my life: Ten thousand people dancing as one. Everyone ecstatic, covered in vibrant colors, smiling and laughing, completely happy and free. There was no distinction between gender, age, race, or class. It was just one massive pulsing, throbbing Technicolor crowd of human beings, celebrating life. My whole body filled with joy. For one split second, I was able to witness the whole thing unfolding, and in that moment I asked myself a question: *How in the world did I get here?*

IN the BEGINNING

IN THE BEGINNING

I T'S HAPPENING!" MY MOM CRIED OUT. HER HEART WAS racing as my dad's foot lay like a brick, pressing hard against the gas pedal of his 1970s Monte Carlo. My mom was in labor. Her breath swelled as she gripped the leather handle on the door, her sweaty palms pushing against the beige upholstery. Her heart was pounding like an 808 kick drum as my dad barreled through the rainbow tunnel, the tunnel now named after the famous comedian Robin Williams. It was a close call. I was almost born on the Golden Gate Bridge. Or so the story goes.

The velocity of my dad's Chevy cut through heavy layers of fog early on that Sunday morning in August. My parents, both in their early twenties, carved a path through the darkness searching for the nearest hospital. Pushing through the two towering pillars of the Golden Gate, speeding past the toll booth into the heart of the city, they found refuge on Geary Boulevard. I was born as the sun made its way over the eastern horizon.

My mom, exhausted and spent, smiled as she looked at my dad. Tears welled up, filling their eyes, as they looked at their newborn child. It was a long journey, through the rainbow tunnel, across the golden bridge to the other side, but I made it, into the warmth and the safety of my parents' arms.

I was a fat, ugly, jaundiced little thing. In my baby photos I look like a pile of mashed potatoes. But my parents didn't seem to mind; they were happy, because I was healthy and I was alive. Later that Sunday morning, my dad left the hospital, went to the nearest church, knelt in front of the altar, and offered his prayers, thanking God for his firstborn son.

After I was born, my parents didn't waste much time: twenty-two months later my beautiful little sister, Melissa, was born, and exactly twenty-two months after her my little brother, Adam, arrived on the scene with a devilish grin. We were surrounded by family growing up; life as a kid in northern California was golden. Our childhood was filled with Saturday-morning cartoons, piles of comic books, baseball cards, outdoor adventures in the trees, and some of the best movies of all time: *Star Wars, Indiana Jones and the Temple of Doom, E.T., The Goonies,* and *The Karate Kid.*

My grandparents lived next door on our left, and my uncle lived next door on our right. Three houses in a row. It was a block of Italians. Because we lived so close to so many cousins, uncles, aunts, and grandparents, I felt a real sense of security and stability. Everything on the surface seemed perfect. Little did I know that the world around me was about to come crashing down. The cracks became clear the night I stayed over at my best friend Dusty's house.

Dusty lived just a couple of houses down from us. We always hung out. We played on the same wiffle ball team, collected the same *Star Wars* action figures, and shared a love for the same Nintendo games. We were two peas in a pod. After school we'd get hopped up on sugar and soda and run circles around the trees in his yard.

We'd imagine we were Jedi knights: I would be Luke Skywalker, and he would rule the galaxy as Darth Vader. Sticks from fallen tree branches became our imaginary lightsabers, and we'd channel the invisible power and energy of the Force, chasing each other through fields of grass, our imaginations running wild, until we'd both collapse, lying in the sun, staring up at the clouds. Dusty took his role so seriously that he even refused to eat with me, because Darth Vader didn't like people to see him take his mask off, and no one—and I mean no one—should ever watch the evil Sith lord eat a peanut-butter-and-jelly sandwich with the crust cut off.

That night, we spent hours playing Nintendo. Nintendo was brand-new, and playing video games at home was one of the coolest things in the world. Dusty and I were playing Kung Fu. "Heya heya"—that sound from the game still rings in my head. But there's a tricky part to that game, regardless of how good you are; there's a moment where you lose no matter what you do.

It goes like this: As you're playing the hero, walking down the hall, making your way toward the big boss, someone comes from behind and throws a dagger at your back. At the very same moment someone approaches from the front, kneels down, and throws a knife at your knees. Two deadly weapons coming from both directions. If you jump you can avoid the lower knife but will be hit by the high knife, and if you duck you avoid the higher knife but will be cut down by the lower blade. Either way it's bye-bye, Johnny.

The moment the hero is struck from both sides, his 8-bit body shudders and falls from the screen as the maniacal laugh of the big boss echoes across the speakers of the television set. Then the letters flash across the screen: GAME OVER!

Dusty's dad unplugged the game. "Time for bed, boys."

"Yes, sir," we replied, filing into the tiny room and climbing into the bunk beds. Dusty claimed the top bunk, while I curled up underneath the *Star Wars*–printed blankets below. "May the force be with you," I said. "And also with you," he responded.

That night, as I dreamt of Jedi knights and video games, something strange happened. It was less of a dream and more of an awakening. As everyone slept, parents snoring in the other room, Dusty's leg hanging from the top bunk, I was struck with an intense feeling. I wasn't asleep and I wasn't awake; I was somewhere in between. I started to feel a pressure forming in the middle of my eyebrows, like a pool of water freezing and solidifying into ice. There was a huge tightness building and gathering inside me. As it grew, it felt like my mind was going to split and break in half. My mind began cracking like the hard, thin layer of an eggshell being pierced by the sharp edge of a beak. The knot in between my eyes grew tighter, and as the moment of impact drew closer, my whole body began to tingle.

Everything seemed like it was slowing down while simultaneously speeding up. I felt big and then small, small and then big, like the cosmic lens of a camera going from a wide shot to an extreme close-up, zooming in and out. And then *snap!* My mind cracked open; I felt a massive energetic swell of awareness, expanding to encompass the bedroom, the house, our town, the coast, until it spread out and engulfed the stars.

I looked down and could see my body the size of an insect; it felt like the genie had been released from the bottle—the clash and crash of two opposing forces, small and big, slow and fast, past and future. It was as if everything collided in that moment, and the intensity cracked my consciousness wide open.

Then, just as quickly as the feeling came on, it was gone, like a subsiding wave being pulled back to sea. Everything reverted back to normal.

I looked around and noticed a stream of moonlight shining through the folds of the curtains. I could see particles of dust shimmering and dancing inside the ray of light as it poured into the room. *What in the world is happening to me?* I wondered. I tried to shake off the bizarre experience. But the memory of that feeling created a lasting echo.

The next morning, Dusty's mom stood in the middle of the kitchen talking. Eating my sugar-coated cereal, I did my best to tune her out. As I looked down into the swirling rainbow-colored bowl of milk, all I could do was contemplate the experience I had had the night before. Then, watching the blues and pinks swirling together around my spoon, I heard her say, "Oh, by the way, can you believe your parents are getting divorced?" She said it so nonchalantly, like everyone in the world already knew—everyone except me.

"They what?" I asked, and just like in the video game, I felt those two knives hitting me from both sides. My spoon dropped into the bowl. Game over. "I have to go."

"You're supposed to stay here another night," she said, but I ignored her. I just left, walked outside, looked up, and stared at the sun. *Is this what that feeling last night was trying to tell me?* I thought. *Was the universe trying to warn me? And what am I supposed to do now?*

EVERYTHING

is

GONNA

BE

ALRIGHT

3

EVERYTHING IS GONNA BE ALRIGHT

T HE NEXT COUPLE OF WEEKS WERE AN EMOTIONAL blur. It was the late eighties, and I didn't know of any other families who'd gone through a divorce before. We were Catholic, and divorce in the Catholic Church was considered a mortal sin. To make things more complicated, when my parents broke the news to me, I also learned that my dad was coming out of the closet. He'd been struggling for years and had finally gathered the strength and the courage to admit he was gay.

As a kid, the fact that my father was gay didn't bother me. In fact, I didn't even really know what it meant. The only other time I heard that word was when the kids at school would say that about another kid if he wasn't good at sports. In my eight-year-old mind I thought it meant being unathletic, but I didn't really care if my dad was good at baseball or not; I just knew that I loved him and that he loved me. The hard part was the realization that everything in my life was about to change. We'd be moving; my family wouldn't be together anymore. I would have to say good-bye to my neighborhood, my friends, the house we lived in that I loved, and the life I'd known growing up.

As if one earth-shattering event wasn't enough, during the divorce the Loma Prieta earthquake hit California. And when it hit, it hit hard. On October 17, 1989, I was at my grandma's house, sitting in front of the TV, getting ready to watch game three of the World Series. The head-to-head clash was between two of my favorite teams. On one side were the San Francisco Giants in orange and black, and from right across the bay were the Oakland A's in green and gold. As the teams took to the field, the entire stadium began to shake, our TV cut out, my grandma screamed, and we all ran for the nearest doorway. The 6.9 earthquake hit the city, and the impact split the bay in half. Houses collapsed, freeways buckled, bridges broke, and fires ran wild.

Both the earthquake and my parents' divorce left a trail of aftershocks. My family began taking sides, and like two giant tectonic plates, both sides were slowly drifting apart. As time went on, I started to realize the gap was getting wider, and in that widening chasm I was getting lost in between.

My dad moved out of our house and into a pink 1950s-style trailer on the top of a ridge surrounded by redwood trees, where my sister, brother, and I would visit him on the weekends. One day, as my dad drove us back to my mom's new place in the suburbs, I could feel a low-level tension hanging in the air. The divorce was taking its toll on all of us. As we traveled along the winding road, I unlatched my seat belt. Slipping out of the constraints, I reached in the back and grabbed my backpack. Shuffling through my school supplies, I pulled out a brand-new plastic-wrapped CD. It was Bob Marley's *Exodus*.

Compact discs had just come out, and we were all excited to be able to listen to our favorite songs without having to rewind and fast-forward like we did with cassettes. Now we could skip right to our favorite tracks. I handed the CD to my sister, who was sitting in the front passenger seat. She slid the thin disc into the machine, and the radio swallowed it, like it was receiving Holy Communion.

The first track on the album was called "Natural Mystic." Bob Marley's voice wailed through the speakers, his vocals rising from the background as he sang the hypnotic melody of the chorus. Instantly I could feel myself starting to relax. The music was altering the atmosphere. It was a good feeling. The song had a way of massaging my mind, soothing my nerves. Bob Marley's voice seemed to make everything better. Even at that young age I understood that music could be medicine, that the right song at the right time could transform the space. It was magic.

The tension softened in the car, but I could tell that my dad still had a lot on his mind. My little brother, Adam, was sitting next to me in the back, his bowl-cut hairdo bobbing to the beat as the music poured out of the speakers. As we made our way to my mom's new house, the third-to-last song came on: "Three Little Birds."

The chant-like chorus had us all singing along, reassuring us. As the words repeated, over and over again, something life-changing happened. My dad's foot pushed down on the gas pedal, accelerating so that we could make it over the hill. Once we reached the top of the mountain, the valley opened up below us, revealing a beautiful vista of endless rolling hills. As my dad turned the steering wheel, navigating the twisting road, his back tire crossed over the pavement, catching a pile of loose gravel along the shoulder. The Trailblazer began to swerve. In an attempt to steer us away from the edge of the cliff, he gripped the steering wheel and overcorrected. The car skidded across the road. My mind tightened. I could feel the fear and panic gripping all of us. As the song continued to repeat, it became less of a feel-good chorus, and more of a life-and-death prayer.

We smashed nose-first into a telephone pole; the pole fell, sending us hurtling down the side of the cliff. The car rolled several times. My sister's hand smashed through the window, leaving huge shards of glass in her right arm, wrist, and palm. Freed from my seat belt, I floated and tumbled in space like an astronaut cut from the line. The music cut out. There was a moment of silence. Somehow, through grace, we stopped. A few more feet and we would have gone over the edge into the gorge, falling to our certain deaths.

The sounds of screams and crying broke the silence. The car was completely totaled, like a crumpled piece of paper. It was the end of a chapter: the divorce had been finalized, and in the wake of the anger and pain of the separation, the destruction was being externally expressed in the crash. The accident happened at the exact halfway point between my mother's and my father's houses.

Because my seat belt was already off, I was the first out of the car. I scrambled up the side of the mountain as fast as I could to get help. As I climbed over the mangled guardrail I raised my foot to step onto the road, and that's when I heard a thunderous voice commanding me, "Stop! Don't move!" As I looked down I saw the live wire from the fallen telephone pole. It looked like an angry snake ready to strike. My foot hovered, frozen in midair. Gasping, I reeled back. Whoever that person was saved my life. Once I saw that there were people pulling over, I climbed back down to help my family. My dad gathered up my sister and carried her up the hill to the roadside; luckily neither he nor my brother had any major injuries. When the ambulance arrived, the paramedics worked quickly to remove the glass from my sister's right arm. The four of us huddled in the back of the ambulance, all covered in dust, as my dad held us close. The doors of the ambulance shut and we sped to the nearest hospital, leaving the wreckage behind us.

Many years later I found out that the accident is what drove my dad to his very first yoga class. That karmic crash that almost took our lives led him to a practice that many years later would save mine. But it would be a long time before I discovered yoga for myself. There was still a very long and winding road ahead.

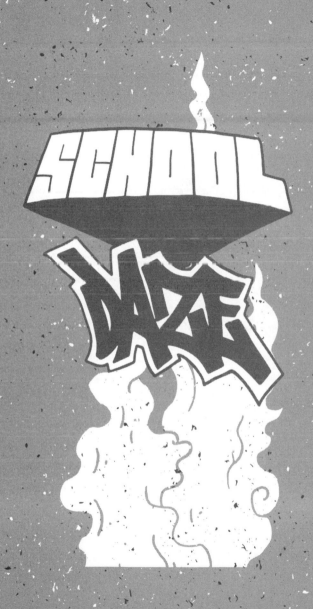

4

SCHOOL DAZE

HE DIVORCE, FOLLOWED BY THE EARTHQUAKE AND then the car crash, left me feeling unsettled; I didn't know what I could rely on anymore. After the divorce papers were signed, I moved to a new school in a new town. It was a Catholic school, and one of the first things I learned at Catholic school was that being gay is a sin, so I kept that information about my dad a secret from my new friends. It was the only time my brother, sister, and I were in the same school at the same time. We all knew the rule: none of us talked about our dad. We held the secret, and in some ways it drew us closer.

Around that same time, my dad and his new boyfriend, Lars, moved in together. I liked Lars. Lars was from Arizona; he had served in the Navy, was a defense lawyer, and owned his own restaurant. He drove a Cutlass Supreme convertible and had a golden-blond mustache.

One late-December day as he was driving home from work he saw a house on fire. He pulled over, ran into the burning house, and after making sure the family was safe, saved every present that was wrapped underneath the family's Christmas tree, including the tree. He ended up on the front page of the paper with the headline "Hero Saves Christmas." He literally saved Christmas.

I was conflicted. On the one hand, the gay people I knew seemed cool, but I was very aware that not everyone felt that way. This became very clear the night my dad and Lars surprised my brother and me with tickets to go see a professional wrestling match at the Cow Palace in South San Francisco.

My brother and I were huge fans of Hulk Hogan and WrestleMania and the countless larger-than-life wrestling stars. We couldn't have been more excited to see the action live. As we made our way through the concession stands, we loaded up on popcorn, soda, T-shirts, posters, and all kinds of awesome memorabilia. The stadium was full of excited families and superfans ready for action, drama, and entertainment. Each grudge match was more animated than the last: huge guys in bright-colored Spandex, with loud personalities, tossing each other around the ring.

As we sat waiting for the main event, the announcer's voice projected across the arena: "Laaaaadies and gentlemennnnn," his words echoed in the air as he introduced the next wrestler to the stage. Loud music piped in from above, electrifying the massive hall. A long-haired, bare-chested macho man wearing a gold cape emerged. As he made his way down the aisle toward the ring, boos began to fill the arena. The lively crowd began to hiss. The hissing was followed by raucous cheers as his opponent was introduced. On the opposite side of the Cow Palace, a real hero stepped forward, his red, white, and blue Spandex declaring his patriotism and pride. As the two men squared off, the star-spangled hero grabbed the mic and began taunting his opponent in gold. "Look at how you walk," he mocked, "look at how you dress. What are you, some kind of queen, some kind of queer?" The crowd erupted with laughter.

One voice began chanting, and then ten voices turned into a hundred until several thousand people in the stadium were chanting, "Faggot, faggot, faggot." My blood froze. I looked at my dad and Lars and saw the dread in their faces. We all decided that it was time to go. After that, I cringed every time I heard that word. The kids at school used it, too, and in the schoolyard they played a game called Smear the Queer. I think most kids didn't realize how cruel they were being, and how prejudiced. The worst part is that there were times I went along with it just to fit in.

Between the divorce, the new school, and the secrets I was keeping about my dad, I had a lot of anxiety. I used to chew the skin on my hands raw, biting my nails until they bled. I always made a point of hiding my hands whenever the teacher walked by so she wouldn't send me to see the nurse. One morning as the teacher was making her rounds, I quickly shoved my hands into the 1950s-style desk to hide my shredded fingers. As I pushed my hands in, I accidentally jammed the sharpened point of a number 2 lead pencil into the center of my right palm. I screamed so loud that the entire classroom turned around and stared at me. I was immediately sent to the nurse's office. The nurse bandaged my bloody palm, and after she saw how ratty my fingers were, it wasn't long before I ended up in therapy.

The only thing I hated worse than school was therapy. I felt like a lab rat, with some egghead psychologist hiding behind a clipboard taking notes as I sat in a box of sand choosing different toys to play with. It's understandable why the adults in my life thought therapy was a good idea. Unfortunately, it only drove me deeper into myself. I turned to sleep as an escape from what I perceived was the cruel world of bullies and overbearing adults.

I became addicted to sleeping, and dozed off almost every day at school. My dream world became my refuge. The only problem was, sooner or later I was going to have to wake up and face the world again. On more than one occasion I was woken up by a Catholic nun slapping a ruler against my desk. My face would be wet with drool, and everyone in class would point and laugh as the teacher scolded me.

The more I slept, the less I cared about school. A few years went by with me totally checked out. I started to fail my classes. And what made things worse was that my failure in school was amplifying the stress between my parents. I knew they were disappointed in me, but I felt strangely distant from my reality and powerless to change my situation.

On the day of my junior high graduation, I ran away from home. Later that night I snuck into the ceremony so that I could say good-bye to my friends. The teachers let me walk down the aisle, handing me a blank diploma, while the police canvassed the streets looking for me outside. I wouldn't be following my friends to the Catholic high school next year; it was back to public school for me. Eventually I completed junior high, thanks to summer school. And since spending summer in a classroom is just about the worst thing ever, that summer I discovered another way to escape, thanks to my new friend Crazy Jimmy.

Crazy Jimmy was the name of a six-foot homemade bong that the older brother of one of my friends built in his garage. I'd smoked weed before, but I never really felt anything extraordinary. Crazy Jimmy was the first time I'd ever really gotten high, and when I say high, I mean even the Transamerica Pyramid in San Francisco seemed low compared to that first space odyssey.

The bong was so tall that we had to climb onto the bed and stand on our tippy toes just to take a hit as two other kids held the bottom and lit the chamber from below. It took several breaths just to pull the smoke up the long, narrow tube. I've never coughed so hard in my life. My eyes closed so tight and got so red that I could barely see the black-light posters glowing on the walls around me. Every little sound became orchestral. I could sense the planets moving and turning, but not just above and below me: I could feel them moving inside me. After that first high there was no turning back, at least not during high school.

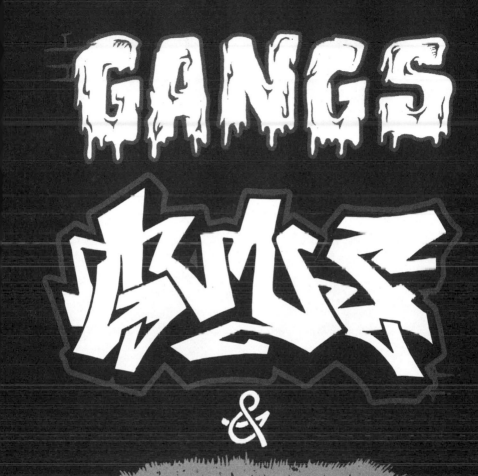

GANGS

&

Grace

5

GANGS, GUNS, AND GRACE

UBLIC HIGH SCHOOL WAS THE POLAR OPPOSITE OF Catholic elementary. No prayers in the morning, no matching uniforms, and no nuns. It was a much bigger school and had a lot less structure. I found it overwhelming. Kids weren't just smoking weed; they had escalated to harder drugs like prescription pills, Ecstasy, and crystal meth. Kids were emulating gang culture as well, and during the midnineties, when I was in high school, violent crime in California was at an all-time high.

One day, after first period, the bell rang, signaling it was time to get back to class.

As I walked through the hall looking for my locker, I bumped into a friend of mine named Little C. There were rumors going around that he was getting ready to fight another kid I knew named Big Will. Little C was a freshman like me, but unlike me he was fearless, cocky, and tough. A blue rag hung from his back pocket, and all his friends wore blue. Big Will was a senior. He played football, drove a Thunderbird with whitewall tires, and was always cool to me. Will and his friends all wore red. I was friends with both sides.

When I bumped into Little C in the hall, there was a fire in his eyes. He raised his shirt and said, "Check this out." I was shocked to see he had a small gun tucked into his belt. As he headed toward the parking lot, a crowd began to grow. Everyone I knew was skipping class to go see the fight. Big Will and a small group of his friends were out in the parking lot. When Will saw the gun, I could see a look of terror in his eyes. He jumped into his car, but struggled to start it. Little C aimed at Will's head and pulled the trigger. His aim was perfect. My jaw dropped as I stood watching the nightmare unfold.

As soon as Little C pulled the trigger he started shaking his gun. *Click, click, click,* he kept pressing the trigger. It was jammed. When he went to shoot, the gun misfired. Little C didn't stop, though; he was on a rampage. He grabbed a huge fallen branch and hurled it at Big Will's car, cracking the glass. There was an eruption of yells and screams as everyone began to scramble. My whole body was shaking; I didn't know what to do. I decided I couldn't go back to class after that. I'd just watched one of my friends try to murder another one of my friends.

A couple of weeks later I was playing Street Fighter II with my friend Joey at my dad's house when we heard about a house party that was happening across town. We decided to check it out. Our usual route to the east side was to hop the chain-link fence, climb down the hill, and then move through the tunnel that ran underneath the freeway instead of walking across the overpass. Along the way we stopped at a gas station to pick up some more smokes, a lighter, and some gum, in case we met any girls.

I sat down on the edge of the curb while Joey ran in to grab the goods. Just then, three cars filled with guys, speakers blasting, skirted around the corner and slid into the parking lot. I could hear the heavy bass rattling in the trunk, like sumo wrestlers trying to get out. I didn't recognize them from school; they looked older. As they climbed out of their cars, I could tell right away they were in a gang. They were rowdy, seemed drunk, and it wasn't long before I realized that they were parking because of us.

"That's him!" One of them yelled. "That's the little shit that jumped my cousin!" I looked behind me to see who they were talking about; I had no idea they were talking about me. I hadn't jumped anyone. Like a herd of angry bulls, they charged forward, shouting and yelling as they rushed toward me. Joey came out of the store right as they ran up. All I remember is the first guy yelling, "Brace yourself, fool," and then the fists: a cloud of angry knuckles from every direction, bone on bone, one after another, breaking against my face, landing on my ribs, knocking me in the stomach. And then, *boom,*

I dropped. I hit the pavement harder than a skydiver with a broken parachute. After I collapsed I clung to the curb, trying to protect my skull.

One of the bigger guys started kicking my head, smashing it against the concrete. I tried to protect myself, but that's when I heard the crack. My nose spilt in half. My hands were covered in blood. The clerk from the convenience store ran outside and yelled, "I called the police, you assholes!!!" They broke out, running across the gas station like jackals as they climbed back into their cars. I could hear the sound of bass and tires screeching as they peeled off, escaping into the night. I never saw them again.

When I got home I gazed in the mirror and wiped the blood from my chin. My nose was so swollen it covered my entire face. I looked like the Elephant Man. My brain was throbbing. I felt like one of the failed players in Street Fighter II; a series of deadly combination attacks left my head swirling with stars. The next day my friends came by to check on me. Nobody knew who the guys were, so there was no way to retaliate. Besides, I'd seen enough violence. I could have been killed that night, and I felt lucky just to be alive.

We didn't live in a bad neighborhood. It was a middle-class area in the older part of town. It was relatively calm and quiet, but on a dark night in the middle of the summer someone was brutally stabbed and almost died on our front porch. It was drug related, and I heard whispers from friends who said they knew who did it. My world was becoming less safe, and I was feeling more vulnerable.

There were two brothers who lived down the block from my mom's house. They were rough kids into selling car parts and stealing bikes. I'd hung out and smoked cigarettes with the younger brother by the creek that ran behind our house. One day after running into him he told me to follow him home. We walked into his room, and I sat on his bed. His room was a mess: old bike frames, piles of dirty clothes, and a picture of a half-naked girl, with the top corner of the poster falling off the wall.

"Hey, can you keep a secret?" he said as he looked through his closet. "I've got something you're gonna want! Check this out." He shuffled through a bunch of old shoe boxes, then pulled a smaller box out and opened the lid, and there was a big, shiny revolver. "It's a .357 Magnum!" he said in a proud voice. "Whoa, what are you going to do with it?" I asked him nervously. "Not me, little homie. You!" He wrapped his hand around the handle, lifted it out of the box, and started aiming it around the room.

My whole body started to get cold. He aimed it at his brother as he walked in. His brother started cussing at him. "I told you not to aim that thing at me, asshole." *These guys are crazy,* I thought. He looked at me again. "I got this for you, man, it's what you need in your life. I'm gonna give you a super-good deal, too. Only a hundred bucks. You get it to me by next week and this baby's yours." I was slightly relieved. I'd thought he wanted me to shoot or rob someone with him.

The gun scared me, but I also wanted to know what it would be like to have that power, that feeling of protection. That week, I started stealing money from every corner of my family's jeans, cupboards, and drawers. By the time the next week rolled around, I had a loaded .357 Magnum in my backpack. I didn't want to get caught, so I stashed it behind the hot-water heater in my mom's garage. Within the first two years of high school, several friends had gotten jumped. I had witnessed one guy get beaten up by fifteen kids at a football game, and I'd felt the wrath of gang violence firsthand when I was jumped at the gas station. I was a shy, skinny kid; when things went down I was usually the first guy to get a fist to the face. I was tired of getting stepped on.

I lay in my bed and dreamt of what it would be like to pull a gun out and make the crowd scatter. My older cousin got stabbed one night trying to protect me at a party. We'd been hanging out at a girl's house in Santa Rosa late one night when a gang showed up and things quickly escalated. I imagined how things would have been different had I pulled the gun and waved it around.

I never really wanted to hurt anyone. I was hoping that having a gun would make me feel safe, but it was the opposite. The reality of having a gun was horrible. It was all I could think about. It made me feel paranoid and jumpy even when it was stashed in my mom's garage. Then I got lucky, because only a few weeks after

I got it, the gun disappeared before anything bad could happen. I suspected the two brothers made off with it; I never found out, and, to be honest, I was just happy it was gone. The weight of fear that the gun carried with it was too much of a burden.

Despite all the horrible things that happened, I always seemed to be able to avoid total disaster. Looking back, I can see it was Grace. First, seeing my friend's gun misfire, then getting beaten up at the gas station and surviving, and finally the stolen gun that was stolen back before I was ever tempted to use it. It felt like there was someone or something looking out for me, like the universe was pointing me in a direction, sending me signs; I just didn't know how to decode the messages. So I turned to the one thing that always seemed to help me better understand myself: art.

LONG ARM OF THE LAW

6

LONG ARM OF THE LAW

'VE ALWAYS LOVED TO DRAW; I WAS AN ARTIST FROM an early age. In elementary school I could draw a perfect Bart Simpson, a really good Batman, and a decent Spider-Man. Instead of working on my schoolwork, I spent most of my time developing my cartoon styles, with the dream of one day being able to make my own comic books. Once when I was around ten years old, my dad and I were walking through downtown San Francisco when we stumbled into what felt like a Technicolor dream world. It was a parking lot covered with the most incredible graffiti murals. Bright washes of hot pink, baby blue, yellow, purple, and light green; everywhere you looked there was color. The place was called Psycho City, a series of parking lots and alleyways close to Van Ness Avenue. On every wall were huge graffiti characters, flying horses, and larger-than-life superheroes. I felt like I was inside of a living cartoon. That was the moment I decided I would become a graffiti artist.

By the time I was thirteen I was already deep into the craft of street art. I loved the smell of the fumes, the rattle of the cans in my hand, and seeing the colors of the paint spread across the wall. The graffiti scene gave me a sense of community. We were a subculture of kids willing to risk our freedom in order to express ourselves. It was rebellious, it was intoxicating, it was dangerous, and it was fun.

I'd fill my bed with pillows so it looked like I was sleeping, then sneak out through my bedroom window to go on late-night street-art missions. I'd been messing around painting some shabby murals and tags for the past couple of years at the freight yards not far from my dad's house. Every chance I got I was drawing, scribbling, or writing on whatever I could get my hands on. My dad always supported me being an artist, and he let me paint my room from the floor to the ceiling, so the walls were always dripping with fresh tags and brightly colored pieces. Friends would come over, and we'd spend all day drawing in our black books, listening to hip-hop, and figuring out ways to create different styles, new characters, and dynamic letter schemes.

When I was a freshman I joined a newly formed graffiti crew called V.C.R.: Vandals Causing Riots. We were a motley crew of renegade artists—mostly skaters, young suburban punks, and semiprofessional drug dealers. My first graffiti name was Menace. I thought my name was so cool. In reality, I was an insecure thirteen-year-old trying to be a badass. I wore my pants so low you could see my entire boxer shorts. To top it off I had one of the worst haircuts you can ever imagine: my entire head was shaved except for my bangs, which were superlong, bleached blond, and slicked back. It was a look my friends called a duck butt. One of my friends, whose graffiti name was Note, had an Afro that covered his entire head. It was so big he looked like a walking microphone. When our whole crew was together, we stood out like a group of cartoon characters surrounded by real people.

That year when Halloween came around, about twenty of us met up in an abandoned lot to party and paint. It was outside of town, and it had some really nice concrete dividing walls. I pulled a can of Rust-Oleum red spray paint out of my backpack and shook it until the paint was mixed. I started hitting the concrete canvas. I wrote my message across the length of the wall, in big bold red letters: I AM A MENACE! My friends watched and cheered me on, throwing empty bottles against the wall as I painted. A light-red mist lingered in the air, wrapping and twisting around me as I walked away from the wall. I tossed the empty can on the ground, lit a cigarette, and then heard someone yell, "COPS!"

The sound of sirens broke up the party. Everybody freaked out, scattering in all directions. A group of us piled into my buddy Orbit's van. I slammed the door, and we all held on to whatever we could grab as the car peeled off. "That was a close one, bro," someone yelled from the back. Everyone started hooting and hollering, celebrating our near escape. "Check this out," one of my buddies said. There were several dozen farm-fresh eggs in the van, ready to become ammo for our Halloween raid. I picked one of the eggs up and said, "I am the egg man!!"

We slid the van door open with the music blasting and started unloading our eggs on the unsuspecting crowd of kids walking up and down the street in their costumes. I was the closest to the door, so I was the gun man. "The yokes on you!" I yelled. My corny joke had everyone in the car laughing. I cocked back my arm, egg in hand, and let it fly. *Smack!* "Oh shit," someone in the back yelled out, "you just hit a cop!"

I slammed the van door shut and yelled to Orbit, "Go man, go!" I looked back and saw the officer huffing and puffing as he charged toward us. Just as the cop's arm reached for the back of the van, Orbit stomped the gas pedal and we fishtailed out of there.

Once we were sure the coast was clear, we found another empty lot and celebrated with beer, blunts, and acid. I decided to pass on the acid; I knew a kid who'd lost his mind on LSD, and was afraid of what might happen. As everybody's drugs started kicking in, I could see Orbit getting pumped up. I watched as he climbed up and stood on top of the van. He called to another kid to get behind the wheel, and then he yelled, "Gun it!" The rest of us stared from the sidelines as the van whizzed by with Orbit surfing on the top, seeing how long he could stay on. They did that over and over again, each time going faster and faster, as everyone rooted him on and cheered.

Later that night, our group thinned out as everyone started heading home. Orbit dropped some of us off downtown. I had my favorite snap-back hat on with graffiti letters painted across the front that my friend Turn One painted for me. Everyone from our crew had scrawled their names under the brim. As we turned the corner, heading up the block, we walked right into the boys in blue. As soon as we tried to turn around, we were stopped by the police.

"What's on your hat, son?" The officer's voice was low and deep. "Is that your name painted on the front?"

"No, officer," I said, shoving my hands into my pockets. "Someone at school made this for me, but I don't know him very well." He stared at the letters. "We're looking for the kid with that exact graffiti name," the cop said. "He has a lot of fresh tags up on the freeway right now."

"Sorry, officer, I'm not sure what you're talking about." I tried to play it off, but he just stared at me.

"Take your hands out of your pockets, son." As I slowly slid my hands out of my baggy jeans, I saw his eyebrows pinch down in the middle of his face just above his nose. My hands were stained with a bright red mist, paint drips all over my wrists and fingers from painting the wall earlier that night. My karma had caught up with me, and I was arrested on the spot. I was literally caught red-handed.

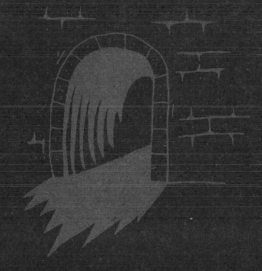

7

GRAFFITI TUNNELS

FEW MONTHS LATER, MY FRIEND KERS ONE HAD A blueprint for a mural he wanted to paint in the Sunset Tunnel in San Francisco. Even though I had already been arrested, and had been slapped with a fine and community service, the lure of painting a big piece with my friend was too good to resist. The N-Judah is a small commuter train that runs through the heart of the city, connecting the Haight District and the Duboce Triangle. A lot of well-known writers painted there, people I really admired, street legends like Twist and Mike Giant. Around two or three in the morning, Kers and I made our way in. We snuck into the tunnel carrying milk crates full of paint, sketchbooks, and cameras. We had our designs planned, and we were ready to roll. As we marched down the tracks, Kers said, "Get ready." There was a light shining in the distance way down at the other end of the tunnel. The tracks began to shake, and there was a loud noise as the air in the tunnel was sucked toward the train.

"Now!" he yelled. Kers's arm pushed me against the wall; there were dark spots in between the concrete dividers along the side of the tunnel. We hid in those little spaces where we'd be safe in the shadows. It was important that we didn't get seen, because if the conductor saw anyone in the tunnel he'd signal to the train authority, and we'd be done for.

Once the train passed we unpacked our gear, looking like bank robbers as we tied our bandanas on. Kers popped the lid of the first can, placed a fat cap on the top, and started going off. "The key is speed," he once told me. The first layer of the piece is always a rough outline; if you've studied your sketchbook drawing, which Kers always did, then you can do a quick rendering on the wall. His pointer finger pressed hard on the tip as a cloud of mist steamed out, enveloping the tunnel.

As soon as he finished the rough outline, he started on the fill-in. It was amazing to watch him work. He was so dynamic when he painted; each move was deliberate. It was like watching a graffiti ninja. Moving as fast as he could, Kers filled the empty letterforms with a thin coat of color using jumbo caps. Huge clouds of off-spray drifted past us. We stayed covered in our bandanas and our hoodies. *Spray paint is so toxic,* I thought, remembering the time the two of us were hitting the freight yards together and I refused to wear a mask, thinking I was being tough; he almost had to carry me home that night,

I was so dizzy and nauseous. But this time I was following his lead; Kers was older and had a lot more painting experience than I did. "Quick, here comes another one!" he yelled out. This time the train was coming from the opposite direction. We were fairly close to the front of the tunnel, so we had even less time to hide.

I slammed my body against the wall, my fingers spread on either side, the cold concrete behind me. I could feel my heart pounding inside my chest as the train rushed by. It felt like the tracks were running through my spine and the train was passing through my body. A huge gust of wind swept through the tunnel.

As soon as the train passed, he went back to work decorating the fill and adding a 3-D drop shadow to the wild-style letters to make them pop. He was almost done. I began to flesh out my character, a b-boy with a tilted hat spitting the words of my tag in a thought bubble rising from his mean-looking face. As I worked the shading, Kers put the finishing touches on his letters. "Only a few cans left," he said. We added our final details, signed our work, and took some flicks for posterity. As we stood back to take one final look at our mural, another light shone at the end of the tunnel, but this time it wasn't the train.

The much smaller light bounced around as it got closer. "Time to go," Kers said. We packed up and started to hightail it out of there. And right as we were about to escape we heard the word that makes everyone stop in their tracks. "Freeze!" I could see the gun. We both froze.

"Hands up!" We dropped the crate of empty cans; the sound of them crashing to the ground echoed down the tunnel. That's when I knew we were in hot water. The man in front of us was an officer from the newly formed SFPD graffiti task force. They had been running a sting operation, and we'd taken the bait. The tunnel was a hot spot, and the city was cracking down. The officer fumed. He was pissed. In his opinion we were lower than garbage. He slammed the cuffs onto our wrists. The metal pinched down, cutting off my circulation. My hands started to tingle, then went numb. The cuffs were way too tight. He leaned his head toward the walkie-talkie on his shoulder and called for backup.

As we sat on the curb the officer dug in, telling us how horrible we were. As he continued to berate us, we watched as Kers's car was towed away behind him. That's when a voice came through the officer's walkie-talkie and cut his lecture short. "We need immediate assistance, over. Do you copy? We need immediate assistance. Drop everything. All cars report to *csssshhhhhhhh*."

"Shit! You two idiots are two of the luckiest SOBs I've ever met." I could hear the call coming in, and it was clear there were more pressing issues than a couple of punk kids painting a wall. The dispatch repeated: "We need immediate backup. Man down. Repeat, man down. He's been shot in the head."

As he put the key in the handcuffs, I felt the blood flow back into my hands. Then he confiscated all our stuff: our money, car keys, wallets, and cameras, but most importantly my favorite sketchbook. That night we couldn't go home, so we ended up sleeping on the street as the San Francisco fog soaked through our thin cotton clothes. We huddled in an alley until the sun came up and the fog dissolved.

Over the years, graffiti artists have been killed, imprisoned, beaten, and robbed, all because they wanted to express their creativity and make a name for themselves. We were lucky we didn't get arrested that night, or worse. Once again the invisible hand of Grace intervened. I was still free, but the next time I might not be so lucky.

After that, I did a lot of soul-searching. I flashed back on all the times I almost got killed or maimed painting: hopping fences, run-ins with the law, stealing thousands of dollars' worth of paint from big-box stores. I started to wonder whether it was worth it. There had to be other ways of expressing myself that were less dangerous and destructive. I'd been freestyling and rapping for a while, writing rhymes and performing and battling at house parties. I loved the feeling of freedom when I opened my mind and let the lyrics flow. The words had a way of falling into place. In some ways, it was similar to painting, but if I did it right, music had the power to reach way more people. So I decided to put down the spray can and picked up a microphone.

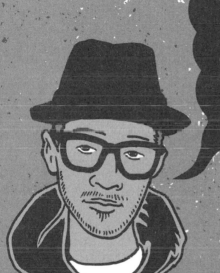

8

ALL YOU NEED IS ONE GOOD FRIEND

THERE ARE FOUR MAIN ELEMENTS IN HIP-HOP, FOUR areas you can specialize in. The first is the DJ, or the sound provider. The second is the b-boy and the b-girl, or the break-dancers. The third is graffiti, or the visual aspect. And finally, the fourth is the emcee—the lyricist or the master of ceremonies.

I loved painting graffiti. I loved the instant gratification of making my mark; I loved that it gave me the feeling of being seen. But I had already had too many run-ins with the law and decided that I didn't want to end up in juvenile hall like some of my other friends. I was flunking out of school. Nothing in any of my classes held my interest, but hip-hop did. Hip-hop became my life raft: whenever the stress levels were high I'd put on my headphones and absorb the beats, lyrics, and rhymes. The focus helped me calm down; the more I listened, the more I fell in love with the art of rhyming. I had tried break dancing but wasn't coordinated enough to really excel at it. So at age fourteen I took my first real steps toward becoming an emcee.

My first rhymes were seriously whack. I stumbled over my words trying to sound cool, and my beatbox sounded like I was farting with my face. But my lack of skill didn't dissuade me. I'd plug my headphones in late at night, listening to my favorite artists, and write rhymes instead of doing homework. Pretty soon, my desire to get good at being an emcee consumed me. I'd work on my craft until I'd fall asleep, and then start back up the next morning. Gradually, because I did it so much, I started to get better. I fantasized about becoming a touring emcee, but it was more of a pipe dream. I never really thought that rapping would be a viable career. In fact, for a long time I kept my music to myself. The only person I shared it with in the beginning was my best friend, Swannie.

Swannie lived just a few blocks down from my dad's house. He was Laotian. His mother crossed the Mekong River while she was pregnant with him, escaping from Laos and seeking asylum in Thailand during the war. He was born in a refugee camp, and eventually along with his family he made his way to the coast of California. We met when I was around eleven years old, and the two of us became inseparable. We were together almost every day during high school. I loved Swannie like a brother. He always had my back, and when someone would talk down to me, or try anything crazy, he always jumped in and was the first to protect me. Swan's a good friend like that. That's probably why I trusted him and felt safe enough to share my crappy rhymes with him.

We'd meet up on the corner of the old service station next to my house and practice freestyling for hours. When I was fourteen I came up with the idea of stealing my dad's car, and we'd drive it all night long around the San Francisco Bay Area, music blasting as we rapped over the beat. We did that for a long time, sometimes every night, always making sure to fill the gas tank and empty the ashtrays so no one noticed. It was a lot of fun until we totaled the car.

One day, my brother told Swannie and me about an upcoming emcee competition, and the three of us decided to check it out. The venue was an old midcentury theater in Petaluma called the Phoenix. It had survived several earthquakes, and like the ancient mythic bird it was named after, it had burned down and was built back up again. It was legendary: Harry Houdini had performed his magic there. Everyone from the Ramones and the Specials to Sublime, Run DMC, and the Red Hot Chili Peppers, not to mention famous local bands like Metallica, Green Day, and Primus, had once rocked out on that same grimy stage.

The theater holds around a thousand people, and that night as I walked in I could feel the energy in the air and the memories in the walls. Cruising past the stairwell, the pool tables, and the concession stand, I walked down the sloped hallway into the main room. There was graffiti covering every wall. The main hall was flanked on either side with huge half-pipe ramps where local skaters practiced their tricks during the day. We made our way toward the back wall and stood on chairs so we could get a bird's-eye view of the place. The faithful were clambering toward the front of the stage, ready for the main event.

The DJ was playing the latest hip-hop from Nas and Wu-Tang Clan to Mos Def and Biggie. He was doing a good job getting everybody hyped and ready. When the host came out, everyone started hollering and cheering, "Let's get ready to BATTLE!" A loud round of applause lifted the energy in the room like a wave washing through the theater. "Let's bring 'em out," he said. One by one, like young prizefighters the emcees who'd signed up for the battle made their way to the center of the stage.

Each emcee stood poised, preparing for the war of words ahead, ready to attack. After announcing each artist's name, the host laid the ground rules. "Once the DJ drops the needle everyone has thirty seconds to deliver their bars, pure freestyle. No written rhymes!" he reminded them. "Get ready to flex your skills. Let's see who can move this crowd. The winner will be the emcee with the most applause at the end of each round." The crowd erupted; they were ready.

I watched like a hawk from the back of the room, taking mental notes as the battle began. My eyes were glued to the microphones onstage being passed around like torches. And then suddenly, as if in slow motion, one emcee, instead of handing the mic back to the host, placed it on the stage. It called out to me, like a lightsaber calls out to a Jedi. It seemed like I was the only person who noticed. My brother seemed to read my mind and gave me a look that said, *Please don't do this.* Then I looked at Swannie. His eyes locked with mine and his face opened with a huge smile, and then without even needing to hear the words, I knew he was telling me, *Go for it.*

I smiled back at him and felt a huge surge of energy fill my body and propel me toward the stage. I pushed forward through the crowd of sweaty teenagers. When I reached the front, I threw one sneaker onto the stage, clutched the Shure 58 mic, and pushed up with the other leg. All the emcees onstage stopped and just stared; the host looked dumbstruck. There was a moment of shock and silence. Something had come over me, and by the time I was onstage and looking into everyone's eyes it was too late to turn back. The theater lights made my eyes squint as I raised the hot mic toward my face.

I had played through this scene in my mind a thousand times, imagining what it would be like to be a real emcee and rock the mic in front of a real live crowd. I would check the mic with confidence. "One two. One two." I would call to the crowd, "Let me hear you scream!" I would get them all to chant to the DJ to drop the beat. Then I would deliver one mind-melting verse after another until everyone's arms would be up waving from side to side.

I took a deep breath in, gathering my spirit, and just as I was about to drop my freestyle, right as the first word was about to leave my lips, *BAM!* I was tackled, hit from both sides by two security guards. Instead of being able to drop my rhymes, I was dropped instead. As I hit the ground, I heard the worst sound ever: *screeeeeezzzch.* The needle scratched, and the music cut out.

"Sorry, everybody!" the host chimed in, apologizing. "The only people who can perform are the people who signed up." "Booooo," the crowd moaned. Before I knew what was happening, I was on my ass in the parking lot as the backstage door of the green room slammed behind me. "Don't let the door hit ya where the good lord split ya," one of the security guards said as he kicked me out.

Swannie was the first to find me in the back alley behind the theater. He patted me on the back, his smile still taking over his whole face. "Good try, buddy. They better get ready 'cause next time you're going to destroy."

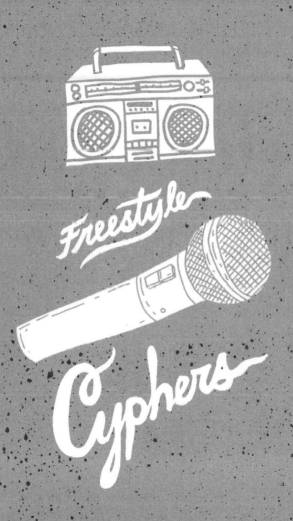

Freestyle Cyphers

9

FREESTYLE CYPHERS

NOT LONG AFTER GETTING KICKED OUT OF THE Phoenix, I heard about a house party happening across town, so I hit up Swannie and we made plans to check it out. The tract house was on a dark narrow street, butting up against the edge of the 101 freeway. The lawn in front of the house was covered with red plastic cups, and I could hear the sound of people making music in the back as we walked in. I stood in the smoke-filled living room, pants sagging, my hood up, pockets full of sweaty palms. The house was dimly lit. Cars and semitrucks whizzed by behind the backyard as a bunch of young suburban kids blew off steam, getting wasted. The smell of exhaust fumes mixed with clouds of tobacco and weed smoke; the whole place reeked of cheap beer. The carpets were stained and covered with cigarette burns.

As I carved my way through the party, navigating through crossfire conversations, hellos, high fives, and what's-ups, I pushed closer and closer until finally I reached a huddled group of hooded kids who had gathered in a circle to rap. The circle, or what we called *the cypher,* was where we gathered to test our skills as emcees. I joined everyone bobbing their heads to the sounds of an overweight kid beatboxing. Hands pressed against his face, he sounded like he had swallowed a boom box. The beat was leaking through the creases in between his fingers. The sound being projected was muffled and dope. He gyrated and bounced side to side, his triple-extra-large Raiders T-shirt sweaty as his spit-soaked hands opened just enough to release the heavy bass of his voice into the empty space in the center of the cypher.

As I looked around I could see some kids making out on the couch as other kids sat around getting high next to them. Alcohol flowed. Most of the guys in the cypher were drinking forty-ounce bottles of malt liquor. Green and gold bottles of Mickeys, red-and-gold bottles of Old English, and the occasional bottle of cheap tequila. Everything was being passed around with a strong invitation to partake. Swannie and I joined the congregation.

The beat changed as, one after another, each emcee took their turn, delivering what they felt was their best rhymes. The rhymes were punctuated with explosions of laughter and applause, or, if they sucked, boos. Most of the rhymes weren't that good, including mine, but every once in a while someone would say something clever, and the entire cypher would react accordingly.

Everyone had their own style. But most of the topics and themes all kind of sounded the same. Most of the kids rapped about guns and each other's mothers. "Yo, your mom's so fat she eats so much bread, she needs a forklift just to get out of bed!" "Ohhhhh." Everyone started busting up, pointing at the poor kid who just got dissed. We were a mixed group of kids, from different towns, different ages, different races, but all of us loved hip-hop. When the invisible mic was passed to me, I began to freestyle:

> The force flows strong through my mind like a Jedi
> The mic's my lightsaber watch me elec-tri-fy
> The whole scene with this supreme rhyme routine
> Illuminate the mental space just like a sunbeam
> Put your hands in the air wave them front to back
> And if you love hip-hop let me hear me you clap
> Off the top of the dome channeling my thoughts
> And when I'm done stop the drum . . . mic drop

I got a couple of claps, nothing major. The next thing I knew, a tall, angry-looking kid wearing a beanie and a black shirt shoved his way forward. He had the kind of face that looked like it rarely broke into a smile. I imagined him scowling in the mirror at night as he practiced looking hard. "Yo yo," he started in. He was like a machine gun of puns. His style was rapid and rabid. As his eyes scanned the crowd looking for people to insult, his sights landed on me and locked in.

> Listen you little bitch
> I'm a put my gun in your mouth pull the trigger
> and click
> Dumb little faggot try to bite my style but
> you just can't have it
> God dammit I'm the motherfucking best
> You're just a little baby sucking on your
> mother's breast
> Look at this guy you can't mess with me homie
> You don't have the Force you look more like a
> gay Obi-Wan Kenobi
> Somebody hold me back before I sock him
> in the face
> This little bitch-ass faggot is a motherfucking
> disgrace

The human beatbox stopped and just stared at me, waiting to see my reaction. It was a moment frozen in time, and then the tall angry emcee blurted out, "You got destroyed, bro!" There were claps and sounds of agreement from the cypher.

His words were like poison arrows. My chest tightened as I felt all my shame: lying and hiding the truth about my dad.

Swannie was one of my only friends who knew about my dad and was cool with it. He pushed forward, and it looked like he was getting ready to sock the other emcee in the face. I threw my arm across his chest to stop him. I thought about how much I loved my dad and all the times I had stayed quiet when people made homophobic remarks. Something in me rose up; I just couldn't let this guy win, not this time.

I rooted my feet to the ground as if I was bracing myself to receive a punch. I took a deep breath, and as I exhaled I just let the words flow out:

It must be hard acting that hard
How many times have you practiced those bars?
Gay clichés maybe you're afraid
Maybe you're scared maybe you're ashamed
Seriously it's okay just be yourself
You don't have to work so hard being someone else
You seem stressed like you just got fired from your job
Maybe we should all pitch in so this guy can get a massage

Everybody started laughing when I said "massage." "Oh snap!" one of the other emcees yelled out. Swannie gave me a high five. As the rounds of disses started up again I decided it was time to duck out. I signaled to Swannie; we said our good-byes and then we bounced.

THE
LAST
STRAW

10

THE LAST STRAW

T THE END OF FRESHMAN YEAR, THE SCHOOL called my mom and me into the principal's office and told us that I was getting expelled. I had gotten straight Fs. I had just stopped caring. I completely ignored my teachers and my homework, and when I did show up to class I was disruptive. After my expulsion, my parents put me in a continuation school. This new school was smaller and filled with a bunch of other misfits like me.

One night a friend of mine from school invited me to go with him and his family to the county fair. We spent the better half of the day playing video games at his house and getting high. As the sun began to set in the suburbs, we met up with his parents, his uncle, and his older brother and walked over to the fairgrounds.

The lights of the rides blurred as they shimmered and sparkled against the night sky. The fair was filled with loud attractions, with stalls selling cotton candy, alcohol, fried food, and tickets for the rides. My friend and I got in line to ride a dark purple UFO called the Gravitron. The ride operator said, "Get ready, kids," in a raspy, smoke-stained voice. As we lined up against the inner wall, the old guy hit Play on the stereo, and heavy metal started screaming through the speakers as he fired up the machine. "Welcome to the jungle," he said.

As everything began to spin, I could feel my stomach bubbling, rising into my throat. The speed of the spinning wheel created a gravitational pull that made our bodies cling to the inner wall. I looked over at one of the kids across from me. His face was green. As the music blasted through the cheap speakers at a deafening volume, we spun like a plane spiraling out of control. I could see that the kid across from me was about to blow. He was trying to hold it in, but the momentum of the ride was overpowering his ability to control his body. As he threw up, all the vomit landed back in his face.

I was about to join him when we started to slow down, the music faded, and the ride stopped. My friend and I stumbled out onto the grass laughing and joking and went to find his family. His uncle found us first, lumbering up to us and handing us a couple of beers. "Here you go, kids. Have fun," he said. I had barely had a few sips when a police officer appeared in front of me with a disapproving look on his face. "Let me see your ID, son," the officer demanded. I was only sixteen, and I was busted. The police officer cuffed me and read me my rights.

The next thing I remember I was sitting in the back of a patrol car being escorted to the jailhouse. That night I was booked and charged for drinking under age. I was thrown in a holding cell for the night. There were two other guys in there waiting to be sentenced. "What are you in for?" one of them asked me, in a not-so-friendly voice. Before I had a chance to answer, his partner, a much bigger guy, stood up. He looked me up and down and said, "I like your shoes. What size are you?"

I had just recently bought some brand-new baby-blue Wallabees. I'd seen Wu Tang Clan wear them and thought they were pretty fresh. I looked down at my shoes, and that's when I heard him say, "Break yourself for your kicks, homie." The two of them closed in. *Here we go again,* I thought to myself. I closed my eyes, ready for the first fist. That's when I heard a loud voice call out from the other side of the room, "HEY YOU!" The door slid open, and the voice repeated again, "YEAH YOU!" The officer pointed at me. "You get one call." *Dear God, thank you,* I thought. The timing of that call saved my ass.

I called my dad, and he bailed me out. He drove up to Santa Rosa in the middle of the night. After filling out the paperwork, I was released early the next morning as the sun was coming out. I ended up with community service, something I was very familiar with. I served my time doing janitorial work at a detox facility that helped homeless people get clean.

That arrest was the last straw. I knew I had a choice to make. A lot of my friends were selling drugs. Some had already been arrested and were in juvenile hall; others had gotten girls pregnant and were becoming teenage dads. After watching so many of my friends fall off, I had to decide if I was going to join them.

I'd failed school miserably. Each time, I would get suspended, expelled, and moved around, only to have it happen again. I'd failed my way out of three schools, been arrested three times. Thanks to my mom I'd heard about a group home for at-risk youth. I didn't know anyone who'd gone there, but the idea of starting over seemed like it might be the only way to shift the downward spiral I was in.

I wrote a letter to the group home, and once they accepted me, I began saying good-bye to all my friends. Later that night I went on a bender with Swannie, one last night to get as high and drunk as humanly possible. The night was a disaster: We ended up at a girl's house in the middle of nowhere, drunk and high on Vicodin. I lost my virginity in the attic, and I remember Swan banging on the wall trying to figure out where I was because my parents were trying to find me. The next morning, hung over and feeling completely destroyed, I gathered up my things and sat on the curb waiting for my mom so she could drive me to my new home. I hoped this would be the fresh start that I so desperately needed.

A GROUP HOME

AWAY FROM HOME

11

A GROUP HOME AWAY FROM HOME

ROM HURT TO HOPE." THAT'S WHAT THE SIGN READ as we walked down the long narrow pathway that led to the main administration building at the group home. It was a long walk; I pulled my heavy bags alongside my mom as we made our way to my new home. She seemed sad, and I imagine she felt like she had failed as a parent. In truth it was me who kept failing, and to her credit, she never gave up on me but kept trying to provide me with solutions.

The group home took a lot of getting used to. It was completely different from my life back home. There were about eight buildings spread across the property, each one housing around a dozen delinquents. I had to get used to the new rules, the new people, the new smells, and the new problems. Certain kids had been there a long time, and they had already formed cliques. I didn't know anybody and felt like a freshman all over again. I really didn't have that much structure in my life before, and was able to slide through the cracks and get lost in between my mom's and dad's houses. Now I had one place, and full-time staff keeping their eyes on me. No more graffiti, no more house parties, and no more late-night joyrides stealing my dad's car. Just school and the hopes of getting a real diploma.

I was assigned a room, an empty space with a built-in bed, and a roommate. I didn't really like my roommate—we had nothing in common—so it took a while to adjust. We all had a list of chores. Every Saturday we'd rotate to see who had to clean the bathrooms. In the morning we'd wake up early, clean our rooms, and clean another assigned portion of the house. Then, before we headed off to our classes, the counselors would come through with a white glove and decide our scores.

Our score would determine our status: If we got into a fight, tried sneaking out, or stole anything, we'd drop to the lowest status, a status four. If our behavior was good and we got good grades, we'd rise to a status one. Status ones could watch TV, drink soda, and make as many phone calls as they wanted. I was determined to be a status one.

Once I unpacked my stuff, I got out my sketchbook, starting drawing, and did my best to settle in. A few days later, Ernesto arrived. He was from the Mission District in San Francisco and was recovering from several near-fatal stab wounds from a gang fight. His parents wanted him to live in a place that was safe, so they sent him up north. He was wild and had long curly hair, fun energy, and a great sense of humor. He was Puerto Rican, and his smile made everyone else smile. We all laughed when he bragged and swore he was the number-one ladies' man. He liked to freestyle, too. We became good friends.

One night he lifted his shirt to show me his scars from the stab wounds. "Yo, bro, can you help me out?" he asked. "I can't reach this scar, and the doctor said I have to put this stuff on it." He handed me the bottle of medicine and I put it on his wound. It looked like a tiger had torn into him with its claws.

A few days later Gabriel arrived. Gabe was cool. He was half Filipino and half Chinese, from the outskirts of Richmond. He was good at basketball, had the best clothes and style, and could tag a little bit. Eventually, because of good behavior, I was able to change room-mates and Gabe moved in. Ernesto, Gabe, and I became a crew. The group home gave me a sense of stability and discipline, and my new friends felt like family.

As sophomore year turned into junior year I was able to get my grades up to a C level. The whole time I was drawing, head down, pen in hand. Everyone wanted me to draw their name or a picture for their girlfriend back home, and I loved doing it. I had drawn several tattoos for friends and was writing poetry. My nick-name on campus was Little Picasso. I was writing a lot of rhymes as well. One of the things I loved about the group home was that it gave me a built-in audience for my raps. A group of us, including Ernesto and Gabe, would gather in the rec room or on the benches outside and freestyle. We'd take turns banging on a tabletop as our drum and perform our poems as everyone listened, nodding their heads to the beat. Occasionally, even the staff would join in.

Then, just when I was getting my bearings, the wheels came off. Some of the kids started smuggling drugs into the dorms. Someone must have gotten caught and snitched. When the group-home administration found out, they started an investigation, and drug tests followed. Everyone was kicked out. It was a huge deal because people had been kicked out before, but never in the history of the center had the group homes been cleared out at once. While I wasn't part of the crew that was dealing the weed, I was smoking it, so I got kicked out, too.

When my parents got the news about the mass expulsion they were extremely disappointed. Back home the drug scene was escalating: crystal meth and Ecstasy were in high demand, and a lot of kids I knew were getting caught up in it. I started to feel depressed, and I knew that if I stayed back home I was going to get trapped in the same old spiral. I had to get back into the group home or I was going end up like the rest of my friends. I started to pray.

I had never really prayed before. The praying we did growing up at church seemed forced, something I had to do or I would get in trouble. I lay on my bed at my dad's house; the walls of my bedroom were a mess of stickers and graffiti tags. What used to seem cool to me now just gave me a headache. I needed a shift, and I needed it soon. So I decided to have my first real talk with God. I said I was sorry for all the chaos I had created in my life; I asked for guidance; I asked if I could please get back into the group home.

Then all of a sudden I heard a voice. It wasn't the voice of God that I was expecting, but it was a very clear message all the same. It was the voice of my Italian grandmother, who we called Big Mama even though she probably weighed only ninety pounds. *God helps those who help themselves.* I had heard her say it a thousand times, and now it was coming through loud and clear. And I believed it was message from God, through my Big Mama, to me.

I got up off my bed and realized that if I was going to make it back into the school's good graces I was going to have to roll up my sleeves and do something about it. I started a campaign of handwritten letters to my teachers, my dorm counselors, and other staff at the school. I started showing up at the center again and again, knocking on doors and begging them to take me back. Gradually it worked, and my prayer was answered. I was the only one out of all the kids they expelled that they let back in.

NOW is THE TIME FOR YOGA

12

NOW IS THE TIME FOR YOGA

I DIDN'T GRADUATE FROM HIGH SCHOOL ON TIME, BUT thanks to the group home I was finally able to get my diploma, even if it was in the mail. Afterward, I moved back in with my dad. In my final year at the group home, I'd been noticing a change in my dad. It was happening slowly and gradually, but out of the corner of my eye I could see him transforming. As most of my friends were spiraling out of control, he seemed to be on a path that was leading him toward more calm, more peace, and more ease. He was losing weight, his presence was getting lighter, he was getting healthier, and he seemed more relaxed.

One day I asked what his secret was. "It's yoga," he said. "But it's not a secret, it's just a practice. All you really have to do is breathe slow and deep, and pay attention."

"What do you mean?" I asked. "I breathe all the time."

"Exactly. Just slow it down and notice it." His voice was calm and steady. "There are some postures you can practice, too, to help still the mind and calm your nerves, but you probably wouldn't like it. It can be hard and challenging at first. It's probably not your thing," he told me, brushing it off.

That was the reverse psychology I needed. I was seventeen, tired of everyone telling me what to do and how to be. I loved the idea that there was a way to relax without all the side effects and messiness of drugs. As we sat in the living room in my dad's house he started to show me a posture. Folding his legs one on top of the other, he sat in the lotus pose. My eyes got big. "How do you do that?" I asked. I tried wrapping my legs in the same way, but to no avail. My body rebelled.

"When's the next class?" I asked.

"Tuesday, but I'm telling you, it's hard at first," he kept repeating. Three times he said that, which was enough to push me over the edge: "I'll be there."

Everything seemed to be leading me to that very first yoga class. It wasn't an ordinary classroom. It was 1997, and yoga was still an underground subculture in America. Even in cities like San Francisco there were only a handful of places that taught public yoga classes. My dad had been studying with a teacher named Larry Schultz, who had just opened a studio south of Market Street after outgrowing classes that he offered out of his living room. Larry taught Ashtanga Vinyasa yoga. In its most traditional form, Ashtanga is a set of sequences that the student learns one pose at a time and then practices six days a week with a teacher, who checks in to give adjustments and corrections.

My dad had found a few friends who also practiced this same style of yoga. In order to keep his practice up in between visits to his teacher in the city, my dad, with the help of his friends, created a simple space tucked inside the back of the barn, inside our family store, where my dad worked. Our family's store, located in Point Reyes, was started in the fifties by my grandpa Toby. Originally, it was a simple hay and feed store and fruit stand. When my dad took it over, he added gifts, an art gallery, a community garden, an organic farmers' market, and a coffee bar.

The following Tuesday night I followed my father's footsteps through the door into an old converted storeroom. It was an open space with old wooden floors, a grand piano in the corner, and a smell of incense that lingered in the air. Before becoming a yoga space, it had been filled with cobwebs, spiders, rats, and bags of backstock dog food for the store. The rustic floors had been refinished and now were glossy and showed the rich warm colors of the wood. The energy in the space felt different: there was a spiritual charge. Even before I started practicing yoga I could feel that there was something special, something mystical, about that tiny room in the corner of the old barn.

I took off my shoes and slid in my socks across the wide planks of old-growth Douglas fir. The low ceiling was held by three pillars that rose from the center of the space. In the corner there was a tiny altar, with candles; a picture of an old Indian man, someone I'd later find out was the yoga master Shri K. Pattabhi Jois; and a tiny statue of the monkey god Hanuman. In a semicircle facing the altar, four yoga mats were laid out: one for my dad; one each for Ron and Chris, the two carpenters who had helped convert the room into a practice space; and one for me. There was no teacher. Everyone knew what to do—everyone except me. My dad smiled and said, "Just breathe and try to follow what we do." I watched and emulated their movements. "Move with your breath," my dad whispered. "I am, I am," I said. He just laughed and kept moving.

There were a lot of push-ups, a lot of warrior postures, and a lot of sweating. Twenty minutes into the practice I was drenched; my whole body was shaking. For the longest time in my life, I'd felt like my body was going in one direction while my mind was moving in another. I'd never experienced the serenity of having every side of myself working together, focused and single-pointed. The only other time I'd had a glimpse of that kind of harmony and clarity was when I was freestyling in the cyphers. In those creative moments when I was allowing the rhymes to form midair, I felt a similar electricity: the energy of being fully present, fully awake and alive.

Each posture seemed to flow into the next, just like my rhymes. As the sequence progressed it seemed to be punctuated by long pauses in downward-facing dog, a pose that challenged every part of my body. As my arms shook and sweat dripped from my brow, I felt the tightness and pulling of my hamstrings. I hadn't stretched in a long time, and my body was in shock. I looked around the room. Ron and Chris were both strong, hardworking guys. When I saw them floating through the practice, moving through intense balancing postures and upside-down poses, it was like watching superheroes training to save the world.

One of the postures reminded me of a move kids used to do during break-dance battles: jumping into a crow pose, an arm balance, and then shooting your legs back into a plank position. I was beginning to think there was something so hip-hop about yoga. I felt like I'd found my path.

The practice lasted over two hours, and by the end I was feeling both exhausted and exhilarated. For the last few years I had become numb. I had disconnected from my body to avoid the pain, the stress, and the difficult emotions I'd been struggling with. In shutting out the pain I had also shut out the joy, and now every square inch of my body was tingling. The heat and the intensity of the practice had dissolved the ice, defrosting my senses. I'd never felt bliss like this before. I was hooked.

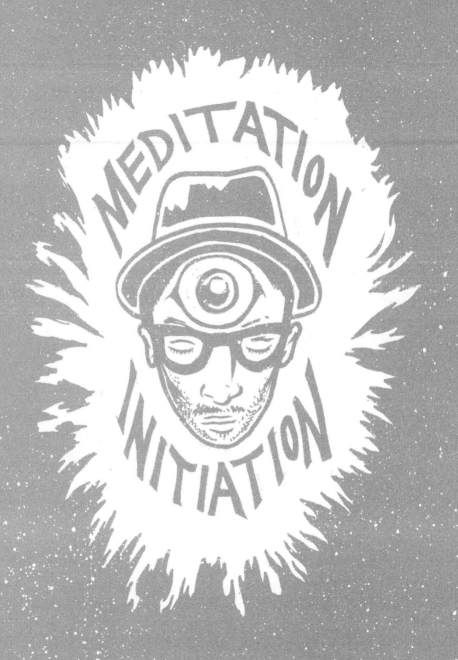

13

MEDITATION INITIATION

I STARTED GOING EVERY WEEK TO PRACTICE YOGA with my dad in the barn. The more I practiced, the more my life began to change from the inside out. I borrowed a huge stack of my dad's yoga books. One of the first books I read was *Autobiography of a Yogi,* by Paramahansa Yogananda. That book lit my soul in ways that no other book had before. The yoga described in that book was mystical; it was all about meditation and experiencing a direct connection to the Divine. I became obsessed; all I could think about was those great yogic sages who dedicated their lives to realizing the Truth. Becoming a yogi become my mission.

I started to live more and more like a monk. I had been dating a few girls after high school but nothing serious. After finding yoga, I decided to be celibate for a while. Instead of chasing girls, I spent most of my time lost in meditation, or alone absorbing more of my dad's spiritual books. My diet began to change: I no longer craved fast food. I became a vegetarian, which in my family was unheard of. I even drank my own pee once because I'd heard that some yogis did it for medicinal purposes. My friends started to wonder what was going on with me, especially my brother. By emulating the yogis I was reading about, I started to have spiritual experiences that were catapulting me into a completely different reality, a whole new level of being.

I started to push all my hip-hop stuff away after that. I couldn't really listen or expose myself to media in the same way anymore. If I was listening to a song and the lyrics were misogynistic or promoted violence, I wanted nothing to do with it. I pressed Eject. I still loved music, but after that first taste of yogic bliss, the only thing I wanted was to learn everything I could about yoga. I became a yoga zealot.

A year into my practice, my dad told me that he was going to see an enlightened master who was visiting the United States from India. I was all in. I wanted to meet a guru, just like the ones I'd read about. I couldn't wait to experience being in the presence of a yoga master. In the past year, so much in my life had changed for the better. I wasn't as stressed out or struggling with depression and anxiety. Through the practice, I'd found a way to help manage my mind and take care of my body. Ashtanga yoga was demanding, and it was pushing a lot of the toxins out of me. Everything was starting to open up: everything started to feel more connected, more synchronistic. The chance to sit and meditate with an enlightened saint seemed like one of the coolest things in the world to me.

The following week, my dad and I drove south into Silicon Valley, where the intensive was taking place. When we got there it wasn't quite what I thought it was going to be. The convention center was like a huge college campus. Thousands of people from all over the world had made the trip to sit with the guru. There were so many people there that they couldn't all fit in the massive hall, so we sat in the overflow room with huge screens where a live feed of the teacher was being transmitted from the main room. *Why did I come all the way down here to watch the guru on TV?* I thought.

Just as that thought was passing through my mind, a beautiful sound began to pour into the room through the mounted speakers hovering overhead. Across the massive screen a silhouette appeared. As the lights rose, the guru's face became visible. Her eyes were sparkling, and she seemed to be glowing. My attention quickly came into focus. As we sat on our meditation cushions, all my expectations dissolved. Her voice was soothing and washed over me until gradually my eyes closed and we began meditating.

As the guru guided us through the meditation my eyes sank into my skull, my tongue softened, and all my senses began to retract. It felt like everything was sliding back into an envelope. The meditation was cosmic. I loved the feeling of diving head-first back into my own being. There was a sense of calm and control, a focused feeling of freedom.

I could feel my legs starting to tingle like they were being stuck by millions of tiny needles. My legs were falling asleep, and my knees were hurting. The discomfort started to pull me out of my meditation. "Keep coming back to the mantra, *'Om Namah Shivaya.'*" The guru's voice was reassuring, like a touchstone. "Use the mantra to stay grounded in the experience," she reminded us.

Om, the sound of creation . . . *Namah*, I honor . . . *Shivaya*, the auspicious light shining in everything.

I continued to sit with the mantra, quietly repeating it under my breath. The mantra had a momentum. The more I chanted, the stronger the pull, drawing me back in toward the middle of my own mind. In the center I could feel a point of light, shining like a brilliant star or spark.

After we'd been sitting for what felt like several hours, the house lights came up. My eyelids slowly lifted, and as my eyes adjusted, there she was again, smiling, like a movie star on the big screen. In a gentle voice she whispered, "Welcome back."

As we continued to sit in the hall she began to teach about yogic philosophy. To illustrate her point, and show how yoga can change even the worst person into an enlightened being, she shared this story. This is how I remember it:

In ancient India there lived a rough-and-tumble man named Ratnakara, who lived his life in the worst way. He spent his days robbing, abusing, and even killing people in the name of greed. One day the man threatened to rob and murder a great yogi in the forest. The yogi looked the man in the eye and said, "Go ahead and kill me. I have no money, I am a wandering sage. All you'll be doing is collecting more bad karma."

Looking confused, the man listened as the yogi questioned his way of life. "Why do you rob and kill?" the yogi asked. "To feed my family," the man responded in a gruff voice. "Go ask your family if they're willing to take on your bad karma." That night in his home, when asking his wife and children, Ratnakara was shocked to find that they disavowed his evil ways. When he said he was doing it to support them, they told him they wanted nothing to do with his bad karma. This realization shocked and rocked the man to his core, and he went in search of the yogi to ask for his counsel.

The yogi felt compassion for the man and wanted to help him, but it was forbidden to teach a murderer a pure mantra. So the clever yogi came up with a solution. He instructed the man to recite the mantra "Mara," which means "kill." "You are a killer," the yogi said, "so you must use this impure mantra to realize the nature of your dark ways."

The man sat and performed the mantra as a form of penance for many years. He sat practicing his mantra for so long that huge anthills grew around him and covered his body. Over time the syllables began to slur; slowly the letters of "Mara" morphed and became "Rama," which is one of the most pure and powerful mantras. Over time, the pure divine energy of the name of Rama began to purify this once ruthless thief. After many years of continuous and dedicated practice, he was able to change his karma, eventually reemerging completely healed and transformed.

When the yogi returned and saw the man, he gave him a new name, Valmiki, and declared him to be an enlightened sage. Valmiki went on to study the great yogic scriptures and eventually became one of the most famous poets in all of India, whose work would be revered and loved for generations.

"So you see," the guru continued, "there is hope for everyone, if you're willing to do the work."

I thought back to all the stupid things I'd done, but the story reminded me that no one is hopeless, and that some of the worst people can become enlightened if they are willing to change their behavior from the inside out.

Beautiful Indian music started to pour into the hall again. The guru began chanting, *"Om Namo Narayana, Om Namo Narayana, Om Namo Narayana."* This mantra, she said, is to acknowledge the great power that sustains

the universe. This blessed energy is what holds everything together; it's what helps us to awaken and realize
our deepest dreams.

As the music grew louder, I joined in and began
chanting with the rest of the massive gathering. The
more I gave myself to the music, the more I could feel
my particles changing. It felt like all my cells were ring-
ing like bells. Something inside me said, *Go to the main
room.* I looked around before slipping out the back door.
I wandered down the hallway, moving in the direction
of the main hall, where the music was emanating from.

I opened the double doors and felt a wave of warm
energy wash over me as I entered the room. There was
the guru, surrounded by musicians and devotees sway-
ing and chanting. I made my way toward the side wall.
The crowd was completely enthralled; they looked in-
toxicated. I just stood there, taking it all in. *I wonder
what she must feel like, I wonder what she's seeing.* And
then as if in slow motion her face turned toward mine.
It felt like she was looking right through me, into my
soul. I could feel the hair on the back of my neck stand
up. I did my best to tune in to her presence. It felt like
my mind was a radio, my spine was the antenna, and I
had been moving up and down the dial and had finally
found a clear signal; I'd finally found the right station
and wavelength.

There was a feeling of lightness, like the weight of
the world was being lifted off me. The chant continued
to grow; the energy began to climb, moving upward

toward a climactic high. Along my spine thousands of little knots were bursting open, tiny flowers blooming and popping, releasing plumes of rainbow-colored pollen. The chant kept growing stronger, the trance deepened, and the whole room started to pulse.

Everyone and everything was humming together, uttering the same syllables over and over again: *"Om Namo Narayana. Om Namo Narayana. Om Namo Narayana."* The rhythm and the repetition of those words washed over and through me, again and again.

After several hours of chanting, a deep calm pervaded my body and my mind. Slowly the voices began to soften, and instead of a rousing round of applause at the end, like I was used to hearing at hip-hop shows, instead of calls for an encore, whistles, and screams, when the program ended there was just silence. Pure, open, spacious silence.

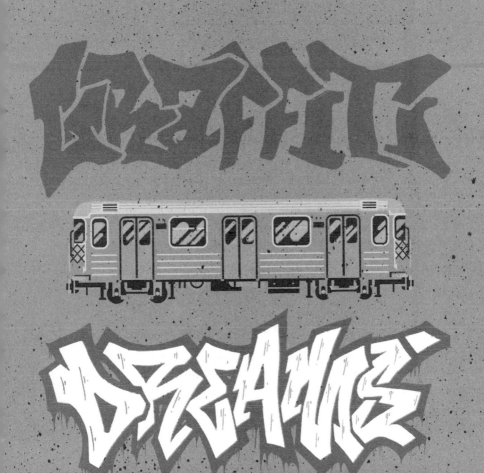

14

GRAFFITI DREAMS

HE LAST FEW YEARS OF MY LIFE HAD BEEN FILLED with so much tension and turmoil. Yoga had lit a fire inside me, and I could feel my practice burning through a lot of my confusion and anxiety. The layers of my old life were starting to fall away. I felt like I was becoming a completely new person. After seeing the guru, it felt like someone had turned the lights on. I was seeing the world in a whole new way. Yoga was reorganizing me from the inside out, and giving my life a new direction.

I was becoming more settled, more comfortable in my own skin, and more confident. I started painting again. My work began to reflect the joy and the good energy I was experiencing on my yoga mat. Now instead of angry, twisted images of demons and skulls dripping with blood, my designs reflected something more spiritual; the imagery became more sacred. My sketchbook overflowed with Om symbols, lotuses and diamonds, pictures of the elephant god Ganesha with his long flowing trunk, and images of meditating Buddhas.

I had a stack of old graffiti magazines in my room at my dad's house that showed street art from around the world. I was starting to feel the urge to travel. I wanted to see what was out there, beyond the boundaries of the Bay Area. I'd never traveled outside the country before. I saved up a little money and decided to go on a solo graffiti expedition through western Europe. The year was 1999, and I was nineteen years old. I bought a ticket, packed up some art supplies, and caught a bus to the San Francisco Airport. I had no plans, no agenda, and no itinerary. I was ready for an adventure.

My eyes were wide as I rode down the long escalator at Heathrow Airport in London. My feet kept time with the hip-hop in my headphones as I navigated the biggest airport I'd ever seen in my life. Everything was fresh; it was like being in a movie. On my first night in the city, I got completely lost in the Tube, the underground subway. Late that night, exhausted and jet-lagged, I wandered into a park with my big backpack looking for a safe place to sleep. A man came forward out of the shadows. He was tall; his dark hair slicked back. He was wearing a leather jacket, and a toothpick hung from his lower lip. His smile revealed his gold teeth. With a thick English accent he asked where I was from. He kept walking closer and closer as he was talking to me, calling me "Gov'nah." As I looked around I could see half a dozen of his friends coming out of the bushes and from behind the trees. In my best fake English accent, I yelled, "I'm from here, and my big brother and his friends are waiting for me!" I turned around and ran as fast as I could back to the nearest Tube station, where I managed to sleep for a few hours until the sun came up.

I wasn't feeling very welcome in London, so I set my sights on Amsterdam. I had heard about Amsterdam from my stoner friends back home, and when I got there I wasn't disappointed. The train ride into Amsterdam was a blur of endless murals, bold bright letters, intricate characters, and rainbow colors dripping from the walls. It was a graffiti dream.

The streets were filled with rows of bicycles, beautiful architecture, and travelers from all over the world. I found a Christian youth hostel in the red-light district and made it my temporary home base. The smell of warm pastries and hot coffee from the cafés filled my senses one morning as I got up early and ventured out into the city. As I cruised on my rented bike through the narrow streets, I could tell there was a real appreciation for hip-hop in Holland. There were party flyers and postcards promoting rap concerts and loud music projecting from the record shops advertising the latest mix tapes. I'd brought some pens and markers from home and designed some handmade stickers. I went around the city slapping my yoga-inspired street art on telephone poles and street signs. Back at the hostel I met a young refugee from Africa who had been living there for several months. He was only thirteen years old and offered to take me around the city. He showed me the cheapest and best places to eat, where to take the freshest graffiti pictures, and where to go to hear the best underground hip-hop.

After a graffiti-filled week in Amsterdam, I said good-bye to my new friend, packed up, and hopped on the next train heading south. I unfolded my map and ran my finger down the page to Italy. *That's my next stop,* I thought. But as the train pushed forward on that long journey south, something was urging me to get off. There was something pulling me toward Luxembourg. It made no sense, because I'd never even heard of Luxembourg, and I had no real reason to go there.

Following my intuition, I got off the train. Luxembourg stood like a medieval fortress, surrounded on all sides by barriers and walls. I found my way to another cheap hostel. While I was checking in, I asked the lady behind the desk if she knew of any yoga studios. She didn't, but when she looked it up on her computer, she found one place and told me they had a class the following day at six o'clock. She wrote the address down on a piece of paper. *Perfect,* I thought. *I'm not sure why I'm here, but I am sure a good yoga session will help to point me in the right direction.*

I set my travel alarm for 5 A.M. It was still dark when I woke up the next morning; I wanted to give myself enough time to find the yoga studio. I wrapped a warm scarf around my neck and hit the local bus stop. The city was still asleep and the streets were cold and empty. The bus dumped me out in a residential district, which seemed like a weird place for a yoga studio. I walked past barking dogs, the steam from their hot breath rising from their mouths in the cold morning air. Finally, I came to a house that matched the address on the small piece of paper I had from the hostel. *This must be the place,* I thought, and rang the bell.

A short woman in a bathrobe answered the door, wiping the sleep from her eyes. "Hello, I'm here for the yoga," I said, introducing myself. She looked puzzled, said something in French that I didn't understand, and then closed the door in my face. A few moments later, it reopened and her husband was standing there, a hot cup of coffee in his hand. "Can I help you?" he asked in English. I could see the short lady standing behind him. "I'm here for the yoga class. Is this the right address?" I asked. "Yes, yes of course," he said. I could hear more French in the background. "But the class isn't until 6 P.M. this evening!" I slapped my hand against my face. "I thought it was 6 A.M. I'm so sorry. Please forgive me. I didn't mean to wake anybody up."

The older woman pushed her way forward, grabbed me by my arm, and brought me into the house. She didn't speak English, so her husband translated. "This is my wife; she is the teacher. Have you eaten?"

"No, but I'm—"

"Let us make you breakfast," he said before I could finish. I was blown away by their hospitality. They introduced me to their kids, who were getting ready for school, and served me warm rye bread with cheese, orange juice, and coffee. After breakfast, they showed me around. We walked to the side of the house where a small garage served as their makeshift yoga studio.

"My wife is a master healer," said the husband. "She'd like to offer you a free session, since you've made such a long journey from America." *Maybe this is why I was pulled to Luxembourg,* I thought. I told him I would love to, and that I'd never had a healing before. His wife opened a door that led to an even smaller room.

Inside there were crystals, Hindu statues, and a table for massage. She motioned toward the table, so I took off my shoes and lay down. As ambient music rose from a small speaker in the corner of the room, I closed my eyes and began to relax. I could feel the heat from her hands as she waved them just above my face. There was a hint of essential oils permeating the air, and the temperature was warm and comfortable.

As I dropped in deeper, I could feel a layer of tension buried deep inside me. It felt like there was a bolted metal door at the back of my mind, and behind that locked door I had stuffed all my uncomfortable emotions and insecurities. Even though her hands never touched me, I could feel her moving the energy around. As the healing got more intense, the door in my mind began rattling and then burst open, releasing a storm cloud of long-held dark energy. I could feel that energy move through my body, and when it passed I felt elated.

The energy that followed was joyful, vibrant, and creative. Symbols and words began forming and dissolving in and around my body, appearing and disappearing like vapor. I saw wheels spinning inside of wheels, rotating like turntables. I felt music in the form of colored mist and giant graffiti letters bending and curving, wrapping around my arms, legs, and spine.

The faint sound of a bell brought me back into the room. I opened my eyes, smiled, and said thank you. "You have good energy," she said in broken English. "You can be a healer too, if you choose." She pressed her hands together, bowed, and then left the room. It took me a while to move. When I finally got up I felt completely refreshed and inspired. I spent the rest of the day drawing and sketching the visions I had had in my notebook.

As 6 P.M. rolled around, I joined the yoga class. It was mostly older women, and the class was taught in French. I borrowed a mat, and we moved through the postures inside the carpeted garage. The style of yoga was called Sivananda. It was very chill, not like the Ashtanga Vinyasa yoga I was learning from my dad, but I really enjoyed it. The pace was easy and slow. We moved through a classic series of yoga postures; *pranayama,* or deep breathing; and meditation. At the end of class I lay back in *shavasana,* the corpse pose, remembering the vision I had had during my healing. My heart felt open and clear, like everything inside had just been rinsed and washed. I felt extremely grateful. Even though it hadn't made sense to stop in Luxembourg, my pursuit of yoga had led me to a profound and transformative healing experience. I thanked the teacher and her husband and made my way back to the hostel. *I'm ready for Rome,* I thought. *Next stop, the Eternal City.*

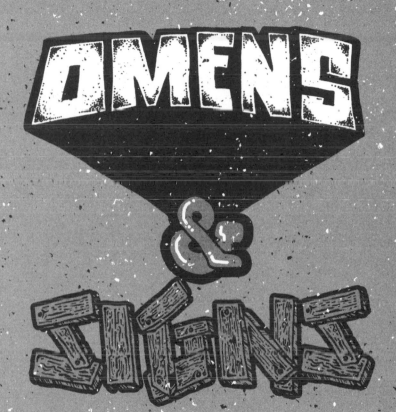

OMENS & SIGNS

15

OMENS AND SIGNS

MY FIRST STOP IN ROME WAS THE VATICAN. I'D grown up Catholic and wanted to take some photos for my grandparents back home. The architecture was beautiful, and the Sistine Chapel was inspiring, but it was also super-touristy and over-the-top. I was hungry for something else.

Walking along an old cobblestone street looking for gelato, I bumped into a skinny Italian man. I could tell he didn't really mind, but I quickly apologized anyway. He smiled and said, "Please, my friend, don't worry about anything." He told me his name was Pietro. He was in his midtwenties, had a friendly face, was tall, wore nicely tailored clothes, and had clean leather shoes. We started talking, and right away I could tell he was a kind soul. Our conversation ended up lasting the entire afternoon. He offered to show me around, and suggested getting out of the city and into the countryside to see the real Italy. The next day we met up and shared a meal at a restaurant that was inside someone's home. I devoured the best pasta I'd ever had in my life, and washed it down with a delicious glass of red wine. After dinner we made our way to an old church. Far from the hustle and bustle of the city, the bare wooden church space was humble and very simple. "This is a place Jesus himself would visit," Pietro said. "No gold, no pretentiousness."

As we sat in the small, empty building, Pietro shared with me his dream of becoming a composer. I told him I was a yogi, loved graffiti, and made music on the side but never really thought I would be able to do it professionally. In his heavy Italian accent, he said, "The muses choose us; if it is our destiny it will happen." Then, lifting his chin, he looked up. "Listen," he said, "can you hear that?"

"What is it?" I asked. His head swayed side to side like he was tuning in to some secret radio station that only he could hear. "All I hear is crickets and frogs," I said.

"Yes, *di preciso!* That's it!" I could feel his spirit come alive.

"You mean you're listening to bugs???"

"Not just the insects," he replied. "Listen to who they're singing to."

"Do you mean they're singing to us?" I asked.

"Not just to us. They're singing to the trees, to the moon, to the stars, and to each other. They are singing in concert with life, the symphony of nature. This is the great orchestra of the universe." Pietro's hands became animated. "We all have a verse to contribute to the universe, and when we are in harmony with ourselves, when we are in tune, we can feel those invisible strings, the sound of the spheres, humming in and all around us. My dream is to help conduct that."

I asked him if he was familiar with the sound Om. "Of course!" Pietro said. "In the East they have understood this truth since time immemorial. Sound has the power to heal and balance us, and Om is the sound of oneness, the sound that encompasses all others. It's the song that the universe is singing to itself." Pietro closed his eyes and began to sing softly. His voice resonated in the hallowed space.

I took a deep breath and joined him. Our voices harmonized perfectly. As we chanted the mantra Om, the sound bounced and reverberated across the wooden beams that lined the church like a rib cage. Everything became saturated in that sound. I could feel the particles in the air changing. As the sound of our voices slowly dissolved back into silence, we just sat there together peacefully, quietly absorbed in the moment.

Pietro reminded me how powerful sound can be, especially when it's flowing from a place of connection and unity. "You could be a great singer," he said. I shrugged and replied, "Yeah, right."

After saying good-bye to Pietro I realized how lonely I was. I'd met several incredible people along the way, but in my heart I was longing to have someone I could travel with, a partner, someone who could share the journey with me.

My trip to Europe ended in Rome, and on my last day I decided to visit a museum that was showing the art of Salvador Dalí. As I was leaving I noticed a group of tourists gathered around a young man standing behind a folding table in front of the museum. As I got closer and moved through the crowd, I could see he was a fortune-teller. He spoke broken English and held a deck of tarot cards.

I placed what little crumpled money I had left on the table. He took the cash and began to shuffle the deck. As he spread the cards, I watched as his eyes lit up. "You have been lonely, yes?" he asked. I nodded. "You would like someone to share your life with, yes?" I nodded again. "You are very lucky, my friend. The one you were born to be with is waiting for you back home. You are destined to meet her very soon."

Then, grabbing my hand, he began to look deep into the creases of my palm. "There is some obstacle, but love will unlock the door." I thanked him. Then, realizing what time it was, I flagged a taxi, rushed back to gather my things, and made it to the airport just in the nick of time. Europe had shown me many incredible things, but I was ready to see if what the fortune-teller had said was true, if love was waiting for me back home.

YOGA
WILL
NEVER
Let
YOU
DOWN

16

YOGA WILL NEVER LET YOU DOWN

WHEN I RETURNED FROM EUROPE I MET LARRY Schultz, my dad's primary yoga teacher and one of his closest friends. Larry's studio, It's Yoga, was located in SOMA, the South of Market District in San Francisco. SOMA was gritty and beautiful, overlooking the water, with the Bay Bridge towering across the horizon and the city of Oakland shining in the distance. My dad and I started to go to Larry's classes together. The scene at the studio was alive with energy, and Larry was at the center of it all. The classes were packed with all kinds of people: all different ages and races, artists, punk rockers covered in tattoos, gay leather guys, cute twentysomething girls, dot-commers, and athletic dudes who would press up into handstands in between every pose. It seemed like Larry knew everyone in the neighborhood, from the staff at all the local restaurants to the homeless guys he paid to help clean the studio at night. Larry was the king of SOMA.

One night after class we joined Larry for dinner. Larry looked at my dad and asked, "What are you going to do with this kid?" My dad said, "I don't know, Larry. Got any ideas?" Larry knew that I had struggled a lot in my teens and had barely graduated from high school. I think it was out of kindness to my dad that he offered to take me under his wing for a while and see if he could help steer me in the right direction. And so at twenty years old I moved into the loft at the yoga studio and began my official yoga education.

My little corner in the warehouse-sized yoga studio was simple, but cozy. I had a ten-by-ten space with a frame-less futon, some curtains, and a single shelf for my family photos, a little statue of the Buddha, and my books.

I'd help out at the studio during the day or run errands for Larry, take at least one class, and at night long after everyone went home, I would sneak out to paint graffiti around the city. I had recently become a vegetarian and had read that in India cows are revered as sacred. A black-and-white graffiti cow became my moniker. I painted that image all over the city, from rooftops along the skyline to the empty lots below.

After those long nights of exploring and painting the city, I loved to sleep in. But like clockwork, at 7 A.M. Larry would stroll into the studio and start yelling, his voice like a lion, "Yo!! If you're a real yogi you better be up practicing!"

As soon as I heard him, I'd shoot out of bed, sit straight up, press my fingers together, close my eyes, and pretend I was meditating. He would pull the curtains back, look into the little corner where my futon was, and say, "Oh good, you're meditating! I'll leave you to it." As soon as the curtain closed, I'd sigh and lie back down.

Larry would go into the main room, roll out his mat, chant the Ashtanga yoga opening mantra, and get into his practice. He'd start flowing through his customized sequence of poses. I could hear his deep yogic breath from up in the loft. I'd roll out of bed, stretch my mat alongside his, and start warming up. "That's it, Lucky," he'd say, calling me by the nickname he'd given me. "The yoga doesn't work if you don't do it." I'd follow his lead, and I did my best to synchronize with him and emulate what he was doing. "It's all about rhythm," he'd tell me. "It's like Johnny Cash says: you gotta get a rhythm, a rhythm and a routine. When it's not dry or robotic, your own personal ritual can set you free."

Practicing yoga with Larry was fun. I had struggled my whole life with discipline and school and authority figures, but my relationship with Larry was different, and his love for the practice was contagious.

There were so many things I wanted to ask him, but it soon became apparent that Larry didn't operate that way. Whenever I asked him something, he'd answer, "What do you think?" If I didn't know, he'd say, "Live in the question. Don't be satisfied with quick answers.

Questions lead us on a quest, Lucky. Seek your own answers and not just what other people tell you. Become the authority of your own life."

His nonanswer pissed me off at first. I was angry because I thought he was brushing me off, or that he didn't know the answer himself and so was deflecting. As time went by I started to realize the power of that teaching, how Larry was training me to trust myself and find my own voice. This teaching would serve to guide me throughout my entire life, and help me to become a better artist, musician, and teacher.

Larry lived by this truth himself; he was an original. His style of teaching was considered unorthodox compared to traditional Ashtanga yoga. Larry had a more creative approach, and at the time it earned him a reputation for being the "Bad Man of Ashtanga Yoga." But in fact he was fathering a new type of yoga that would later be one of the most popular styles, known as Vinyasa or Flow.

One day after class, while everyone was chilling out in the studio, I got to hear the story behind his unique method of teaching. Larry told us, "When I was a young yoga teacher, after studying and practicing with my guru, Shri K. Pattabhi Jois, I received a phone call. In those days there was no Internet, so we ran ads in the yellow pages, and apparently someone saw my ad for yoga, and when I answered, I heard the craziest thing I'd ever heard in my life. It was the Grateful Dead! The Dead were touring, and they were looking to do some yoga on the road. I hung up the phone thinking it was some kind of practical joke. But the very next day I followed up, just in case. Before you know it, I was in a hotel room with one of the most famous rock bands in the history of America.

"I was a huge fan of the Grateful Dead, so I was nervous. When the day came to meet up with the band, I led them through the primary series of Ashtanga yoga, just like my teacher taught it to me. It was a rigorous routine; the sequence of postures can be grueling even for advanced yogis. The next day I found out the members of the band weren't feeling the discipline; in fact, they hated it. It was too intense, too rigid. I had a talk with the guitar player, Bob Weir. He said, 'We can't do this, man. You have to teach us something we can do on the road.' So I went back into the lab and started to experiment on myself with different routines, trying to find the perfect combination of postures and sequences. It was through that process that I was able to develop a flow that was more accessible, more fluid, and more fun."

Larry continued, "The next time we met up at the hotel, we rolled out our mats like magic carpets, and off we went. 'That's it, man,' Bob Weir said. I turned to Bob and said, 'What should we call it?' Bob took one look at me, and without skipping a beat, he said 'The Rocket!' I was stunned. 'Why should we call it the rocket?' I asked. 'Because it gets you there quicker, man!' Everyone started laughing, and after that they started calling me the Rocket Man."

When Larry finished his story, I gave him a high five. "Right on, Rocket Man!" I was surprised to learn that day the underground history of how modern Vinyasa yoga began its long, strange trip into the American mainstream. Even to this day most students and teachers don't know that it was in large part thanks to Larry and his time with the Grateful Dead. I'm so grateful for those early years with Larry. Thanks to him, I learned so much about the heart and soul of the practice.

One of the characters who used to frequent Larry's studio was a guy in his midtwenties with a shaved head and a yoga mat with the word *SLAYER* scrawled across the top in huge hand-drawn black letters. He came every day to Larry's 4:30 P.M. class and practiced the whole time with his headphones on. When that class ended and everyone else lay down for resting pose, he just kept going, right on through to the 6 P.M. class, and didn't stop! Over three straight hours of yoga. When I asked Larry about him, he said the guy was getting off heroin. Larry was okay with him doing whatever he needed to do to keep practicing yoga. Moments like that showed me what kind of teacher Larry was: he accepted all of us exactly as we were.

One morning after practicing together, Larry looked directly into my eyes and asked me the most important question anyone had ever asked me: "What's your soul's purpose?"

"My soul's purpose?" I was speechless.

"Why are you here?" he asked.

I had no idea how to answer. "Well, I love yoga, but I'm not really sure what my soul's purpose is." Larry looked at me and smiled. "If you are serious about yoga, if you really commit to it, yoga will never let you down. I'm telling you right now, it will take you to places you've never dreamt of. Take it from me," he said. "Yoga will open doors that you never even knew existed." I'd been practicing yoga for only a couple of years, but deep down I knew that what he was saying was true.

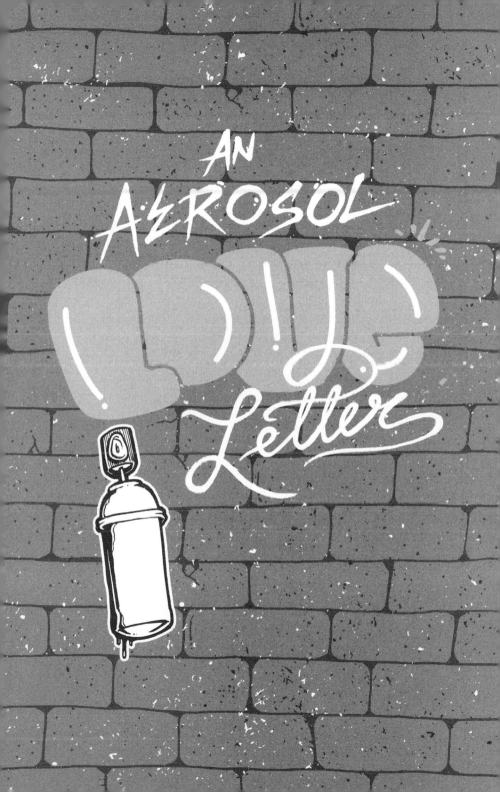

17

AN AEROSOL LOVE LETTER

I HAD BEEN PRACTICING YOGA FOR THREE YEARS WHEN Larry started encouraging me to take the teacher training. I really wasn't interested in becoming a teacher. "Even if you don't want to teach," he said, "it will help you develop your voice, and it'll be a great way to learn more about yoga." I realized he was right, so I signed up for the program. Anything to spend more time with Larry and practice more yoga sounded good to me.

The day before our training started, I was having lunch with Larry at the studio. Larry was telling me stories about his travels, studying with different teachers, and how yoga changed his life. His back was to the door, and as he was talking a young woman appeared in the entryway.

She had dark hair, freckles, and two mismatched socks pulled up to her knees. She smiled, and a warm feeling washed over me. Larry looked at me, lifted his eyebrow, then turned around to see who it was. "Amanda!" he called out. "How are you, dear?"

"I'm very good, Larry." Her voice was soft and sweet.

"I'm so happy you're here!" he said. "Hey, Lucky, this is Amanda. She's going to be taking the teacher training, too." We said hello and made some small talk. I was having trouble concentrating on the conversation. There was something about her face and her voice that felt so familiar. Then, out of the blue, Larry started talking about couples that had met at his yoga studio. "It happens all the time," he said. "People come here to the studio and start practicing yoga, and the next thing you know they are falling in love, getting married, and opening their own yoga studios." Larry's voice was filled with enthusiasm. As I looked over at Amanda, a little voice inside me said, *She's the one.*

Later that night as I hung out alone in the studio I remembered what the fortune-teller had said to me in front of the art museum in Rome. "The one you were born to be with is waiting for you back home." As I lay on my futon staring up at the stars through the window above the loft, all I could think about was Amanda's face.

The next day we all met in the main practice room and began our training. We gathered in a circle, and Larry asked us to go around and introduce ourselves and say a few words about what had brought each of us to yoga, and what our purpose was for taking the teacher training. We were a group of twenty-six students. I was one of only two guys in the training, and at twenty years old I was the youngest. As each person spoke I realized that almost everyone had come to yoga to help heal some trauma in their life.

When it was Amanda's turn to speak, tears welled up in her eyes. She found yoga after being diagnosed with a rare autoimmune disease, and on the same day she was diagnosed, one of her best friends committed suicide. "Yoga got me through the hardest part of my life," she said, and now she was here to learn how she could help others. Her story moved me. I felt some kind of invisible connection with her and wanted to get to know her more.

As our group settled in, Larry began to unpack the basic elements of a Vinyasa yoga class. We learned about *ujjayi pranayama,* or the victorious breath; *asanas,* or the postures; and *bandhas,* the energetic locks that help to contain our energy. He also emphasized the importance of *drishti,* the one-pointed vision that helps to focus the mind. My one-pointed vision was on Amanda: I kept staring at her, waiting for her to look at me— which she never did. As Larry unfolded the philosophy and offered his teaching tips, he had us break up into smaller groups, and I always made a point of being in Amanda's.

As I got to know everybody in the group, I found out Amanda and I had a lot in common. We were both the products of divorced families and were both really close to our grandparents, who had helped take care of us when our parents split up. She was also an artist and loved listening to old-school jazz. The deepest connection we shared, though, was our love of yoga. The intensity of the training was opening us up not just physically but spiritually, and it was reassuring to have someone to share these new experiences with.

We met every day, practiced with Larry, observed classes, and in between studied poses, anatomy, sequencing, and philosophy. For someone who was never very interested in school, I was completely engrossed, soaking it up like a sponge.

In the weeks that followed Amanda and I were almost inseparable. We spent all our lunch breaks together sharing inside jokes, laughing about someone who farted in class, wandering the alleys around the studio looking for cool murals, or visiting the record shop around the corner to listen to music. She was by far the coolest girl I had ever hung out with. I used to make her little gifts, handmade cards with poems and drawings. With every passing day, I felt like the prediction of the fortune-teller in Rome was coming true and that for sure Amanda was the person I was meant to be with. One night I decided I would make her something really special to show her how I felt.

Just before the training ended, I asked Amanda to stay after class and told her I had something I wanted her to see. "Follow me," I said, and started to climb up the cubby shelves at the back of the studio. She looked at me like I was crazy. Above the shelves was a row of windows that tilted open and led to the rooftop of the building. I had to do some pretty weird yoga contortions to climb through them. When I got outside, I stuck my head back in and said, "Come on!"

"I'm not going out there," Amanda said. "It's danger-ous!" The back of the building looked down on a series of narrow alleys that were usually filled with homeless people smoking crack or shooting heroin. "Trust me, you're gonna wanna see this," I said. Finally, she con-sented, and I helped pull her up through the windows. Once we were both outside in the open air, I pointed at the side of the building and said, "Check it out!"

Amanda's head lifted, and as her eyes adjusted to what she was seeing, I could see her face light up. "Oh my God! Is that me?" Her voice spiked with joy. "Yeah," I said. It was a giant graffiti portrait: Her face painted as high as my arms could reach—ponytail, freckles, bangs, and all. A soft Mona Lisa smile, and two beautiful lotus eyes. "I love it!" she said. My heart swelled as I saw the emotion in her face, but then she looked away and low-ered her eyes. "I have to tell you something," she whis-pered. "What is it?" I asked nervously, reaching for her hand. She pulled away. "I'm married," she said.

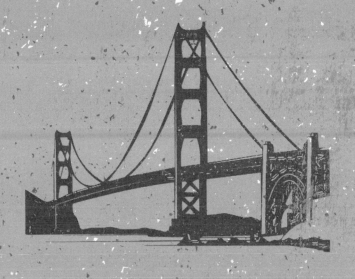

GOLDEN GATE *Bridge*

18

GOLDEN GATE BRIDGE

HE TEACHER TRAINING ENDED AND I DIDN'T SEE Amanda for a long time. I was a mess. I couldn't stop thinking about her. In my heart I was sure she was my soul mate. Nothing made sense to me anymore. Then one night she came to class and told me she needed to talk and wanted to take me somewhere. I agreed, and she said she would pick me up at the studio at 4:30 the next morning.

I had no idea why we needed to meet so early, but I didn't ask any questions and was ready and waiting for her in the dark outside the studio when she drove up. We cut a path through the dark streets of the city until finally we arrived at the parking lot at the base of the Golden Gate Bridge.

The sun was just beginning to rise. The bridge reached across the water like an outstretched arm. Its two towers rose like the spires of a temple, and the soft gray fog billowing around and through the dark orange railings made it seem like a dream. "Will you walk with me?" she asked. The morning air was cold against my face. We both wore sweatshirts and put our hoods up as we began our journey across the bridge.

We were quiet for a long time. I struggled to find the right words to break the silence. "Isn't it beautiful?" I said as I looked at her. "The city, I mean." "It's incredible," she said. When we got to the middle of the bridge we stopped. The city shone in the distance like a postcard. A swarm of sailboats blew past Alcatraz Island as flocks of seagulls created patterns in the pale blue sky. When we turned to face the other direction, we could see the green cliffs of Marin and the Pacific Ocean stretching around them like a curved infinity pool. Then Amanda turned to face me, looked into my eyes, and revealed her true feelings. She told me that since we met it had been both the most amazing and most confusing time in her life. "I don't know what to do," she said, tears welling up in her eyes. "I am falling in love with you, but I don't want to hurt my husband. He is a good person and has done nothing wrong."

Standing there on the bridge, I felt time slowing down to a crawl. As I listened to her words I felt like I had left my body and was looking at us from a distance, two tiny figurines against an epic backdrop of sea and sky.

I held her close. I was elated to learn that she had feelings for me, too, but had no idea what to do next. *Ahimsa,* or nonharming, as we learned in our teacher training, was one of the core tenets of yoga. Standing there on the bridge, we realized there was no course of action we could take that would be free from harming someone. I closed my eyes, asking for guidance. That's when I heard Amanda whispering a prayer. *If we are meant to be together, may we create the least amount of harm for everyone involved; may our relationship be for the benefit of all beings.*

We walked back to the car, and on the drive back to *It's Yoga* we decided it would be best if we didn't see each other for a while so she could get clear about her marriage. My birthday was coming up in a couple of months. I told her, if she decided she wanted to be with me, and to walk this path together, to show up to my birthday party at my dad's house. If she didn't show up, I would know that it wasn't meant to be, and I would do my best to move on. It was a difficult decision, but I knew it was the right thing to do, and so we said good-bye.

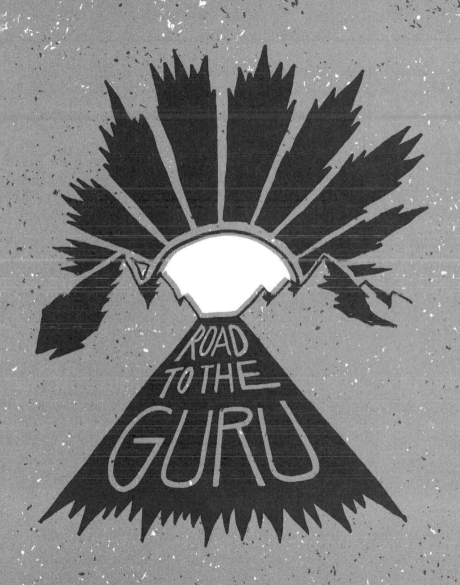

19

ROAD TO THE GURU

THE NIGHT OF MY TWENTY-FIRST BIRTHDAY PARTY finally arrived. Surrounded by family and some of my oldest friends, I waited anxiously, staring at the clock, wondering whether or not Amanda was going to show up. Food was served, drinks were poured, and as the hours passed I found myself looking down at my watch every few seconds. I hadn't heard from Amanda in months. *She's not coming,* I thought. *That's it.* I tried to give my attention to everyone at the party, doing my best to be happy and celebrate what was supposed to be a huge turning point in my life, but in the back of my mind all I could hear was the sound of the clock ticking. If she didn't show up soon I would have to blow out the candles, and with them the hope of us being together.

As we sat around eating cake, my dad handed me an envelope. Inside was a folded flyer for a weeklong intensive with Shri K. Pattabhi Jois, the guru of Ashtanga yoga.

The event was taking place in Encinitas, north of San Diego, the next day. "Happy Birthday," my dad said as I opened it. I was thrilled. I had heard from friends at the studio that Pattabhi was coming to America, and everyone was excited to study with our teacher's teacher, the great yoga master from India. "I reserved two spots," my dad said, "one for you and one for—" Just then, I heard a noise from the front of the house. I ran to the door, turned the knob and opened it, but no one was there. My heart sank.

As I went to close the door I heard a soft voice behind me. "Is it too late? Did I miss the party?" It was Amanda! I wrapped my arms around her and lifted her up off the ground. When we went back inside, we learned that my dad had registered both of us for the intensive. He had known about our friendship, and somehow he had used his fatherly intuition to know that she would show up to my party.

"The intensive starts tomorrow," my dad said. "But you should probably rest and drive down in the morning." I was ecstatic. I was on the happiest natural high of my life, and felt like I could do anything. I turned to Amanda. "I think we should go for it. If we drive all night we can be there for the first class."

That night after everybody left, we made a pot of coffee, I grabbed my yoga mat, and we packed a few things into Amanda's car. We waved good-bye to my dad and sister and headed east through Oakland until we found ourselves on Interstate 5. The I-5 is a seemingly endless strip of pavement that runs through the center of California like a spine. It would take us about eight or nine hours of nonstop driving through the night to get all the way down to Encinitas. We were determined to be there for the first session.

It was when we were alone in the car on that long stretch of highway that Amanda shared with me that she was getting a divorce. She was sad. She told me how hard it had been, how she and her husband had tried counseling but in the end had realized that they were on different paths. They had married young and didn't have any kids or joint assets, so she had filed the paperwork herself at the courthouse.

I could tell that Amanda was emotionally exhausted. I told her to rest while I took another turn behind the wheel. She curled up into the corner of her seat, using my sweatshirt as a pillow, and fell asleep. I slid a fresh cassette into the stereo. It was a recording of classical Indian ragas. The music was so peaceful as we made our way along the dark highway. As the hypnotic melodies swirled, my eyes started to grow heavy. The sound of a blaring horn woke me up; I had been drifting into the oncoming lane. I rolled down the window for fresh air. Blinking hard and opening my eyes wide, I tried to refocus on the road ahead. I turned up the music and started rapping to it as a way to keep myself awake.

The next time I opened my eyes I realized I had fallen asleep at the wheel. I was in the fast lane going about eighty miles an hour. I panicked, slamming on the brakes to avoid ending up in the wrong lane. The car spun out of control. We skidded off the road. Amanda woke up in the middle of it all; there was a look of confusion and fear in her eyes. Everything went into slow motion: for a moment we were weightless and suspended in space. And then the crash. We smashed through a metal fence, flipping the car and rolling until finally we landed in an empty field. The front end of the car was destroyed.

The car landed on the driver's side, so when I reached up to unbuckle Amanda's seat belt, she fell into my arms. I was in shock. I looked down to check that all our arms and legs were intact and there were no major injuries. The car engine had stopped, but the meditation music was still playing. In the stillness of the early morning there was no one around. The roads were empty. When we climbed out of the mangled car we realized we were in a field of wildflowers. The sky was slowly shifting from dark purple to blue; looking up, I could still see a few faint stars. The field became gold and orange as the darkness dissolved in front of our eyes. Amanda looked at me. "Is this heaven?"

There was an honest-to-God moment when neither of us knew if we were alive or if we had died. Holding each other in that field of flowers, as the Indian music played and the sun rose in front of us, it felt like we were in a celestial realm. The car was totaled, but somehow through Grace both of us were okay. This would be the third time in my life I walked away from a major car crash unharmed. I was beginning to think Larry was right in giving me the nickname Lucky.

A woman driving a semitruck pulled over and told us she'd phoned for help. The police came, and after a report was made we asked the cop to take our picture. The officer asked if we were on drugs because we were smiling so much. We were so happy to be alive and to be together that nothing else, including a totaled car, seemed to matter. As the officer took our photo in front of Amanda's destroyed vehicle, we smiled, throwing our arms in the air like we'd won the lotto.

A tow truck gave us a ride to the nearest rental-car agency. Both of us were covered in dust, with little pieces of gravel still in our hair. It's a wonder the rental-car place even let us leave the lot, but nothing was going to stop us from practicing with the guru.

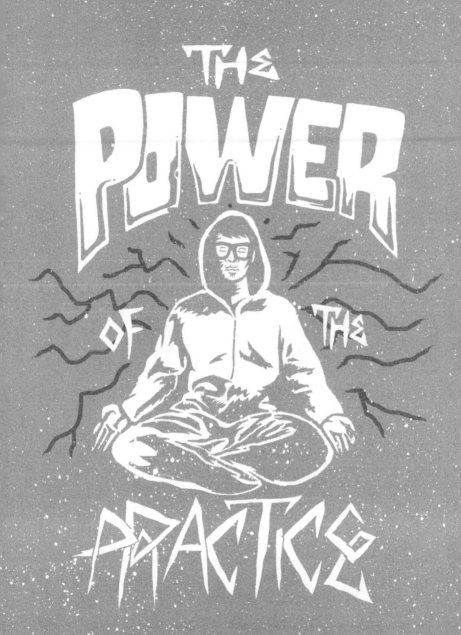

20

THE POWER OF
THE PRACTICE

I T WAS NO SMALL MIRACLE THAT WE ARRIVED JUST IN
time for the start of the first class. We ended up in
the front row in a room of over four hundred yogis
standing at attention awaiting the first instruction from
the master teacher. Pattabhi Jois, or Guruji, as his students affectionately call him, shuffled into the room,
standing in front of us like a drill sergeant. Guruji was
a short, stocky Indian man whose presence demanded
focus and respect.

We chanted the invocation together, followed by the
mantra *Om* signaling the beginning of the practice.
"Inhale up!" Guruji's voice echoed throughout the gymnasium. I threw my arms up with feeling. I was still a
little dazed and delirious from the crash, my neck hurt,
and I was probably suffering from whiplash, but I was
so incredibly stoked and happy to be practicing yoga
with Guruji that it didn't matter. As I dropped into the

rhythm of the breath, I started to move in time with the overflowing gym filled with mostly super-athletic southern Californian surfer-types.

This was not your grandma's yoga. Postures came in like sets of waves. As Guruji called them out, Amanda and I cycled through the practice, like synchronized swimmers. One push-up after another, breaking through mental walls and pushing our bodies through the lingering residue of the car accident. An hour and fifteen minutes later, feeling sweaty, exhilarated, and realigned, we started our finishing postures. Throwing my legs over my head into a plough pose, I remembered Larry telling me the story of how Pattabhi Jois found his way to yoga.

As a young boy Pattabhi Jois was extremely poor. One of nine kids, he was the son of a Brahmin priest and astrologer. When he was twelve he witnessed a yoga demonstration at a middle school, led by the famous yogi Shri T. Krishnamacharya. Pattabhi was so inspired by what he saw that he asked Krishnamacharya to become his guru. For the next two years, Pattabhi practiced every day before going to school. He'd walk over three miles each way to practice with his teacher. When he was fourteen he ran away from home with two rupees in his pocket on a quest to deepen his knowledge. He found his way to Mysore. Around that same time the maharaja, or king, of Mysore became ill and sent for Pattabhi's teacher, Krishnamacharya. The king was cured through yoga, and because he was so grateful, he established a center for yogic learning and installed the great yogi Krishnamacharya as the director. Pattabhi Jois would continue to study with his teacher at the new center, and would go on to become one of the most well-known ambassadors of yoga in the world.

Here we were, practicing with this legendary yogi. He was eighty-five years old, yet his energy was unstoppable. He was strong and alert, and his presence carried a spiritual power. *I hope I can be as healthy as he is at that age,* I thought. "Exhale!" Pattabhi's voice broke through my thinking mind, keeping me focused on the task at hand.

As we approached the final postures, my body was starting to feel better again. After twenty-five slow, deep breaths in a headstand, there was one final challenge. A pose called *utpluthih.* I folded my legs into full lotus, pressed my palms flat against the floor, and lifted my whole body up and off the ground. Guruji was counting to fifteen, but kept losing track of his count. I think he did it on purpose to see if we could strengthen our resolve. My muscles trembled from the exertion. I looked around as yogis were dropping like flies left and right. Finally, after what felt like forever I placed my lotus back on the ground, lifted myself up, and moved through one final transition, floating back into the last push-up, the last upward-facing dog and downward-facing dog.

I jumped through, lay down, and took rest in the corpse pose. As I began to relax I could feel the surface of my body dissolving. There was a huge groundswell of bliss just below the layer of my thinking mind. As I surrendered to the undercurrent, I could feel my mind soften—no longer clinging, trying to calculate, strategize, and organize the world around me. Everything became quiet and still. There was a deep feeling of abiding peace.

After one of the most satisfying *shavasanas* of my life, I could sense the other yogis in the gymnasium slowly beginning to stir. The air sparkled with a collective feeling of joy. Before long everyone was moving again. I felt my mind kicking back into gear. I rolled to the right side in a fetal position, taking a moment to soak in the experience. Moving slowly like I was underwater, I made my way back up, into a comfortable seat. Amanda was getting up at the same time. We rolled up our mats and joined the procession of grateful yogis lining up to thank Guruji. When it was our turn, as the custom in India goes, we humbly folded our hands, bowed, and touched his feet. This ancient gesture, I later learned, is a way of respecting our elders and our teachers. As we said our thank-yous, Guruji smiled, looked at both of us, and said, "When are you coming to visit me in India?"

JOURNEY

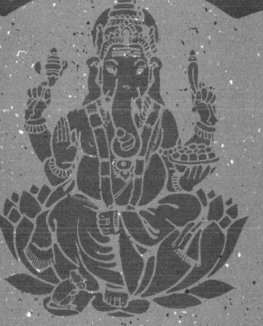

TO
INDIA

21

JOURNEY TO INDIA

SIX MONTHS AFTER MEETING PATTABHI JOIS IN Encinitas, Amanda and I started to plan our pilgrimage to India. We researched different ashrams, holy temples, and sacred monuments, where to go to meet living saints, and the best places to experience the magic and mysticism of India. At the center of our trip would be a three-month study period in Mysore, where Pattabhi Jois had his teaching institute. We saved up some money, and thanks to the generosity of Amanda's dad, who gave us his frequent flyer miles, we were able to get two round-trip tickets to India.

The night of our departure, we showed up for the flight fully prepared. We had eye pillows, neck cushions, rosewater misters, Ayurvedic oils to keep our noses lubricated, homeopathic jet-lag pills, earbuds, and everything else two yogis might need for a twenty-plus-hour journey across the sky. We settled into our tiny economy seats at the back of the plane, and I said a few mantras as the plane gathered speed down the runway and lifted into the air. Looking out the window, I watched as my hometown got smaller behind us and the rest of the world opened in front of us.

Halfway through our flight, I put my Lonely Planet book away, closed my eyes, and fell into a dream. I have a habit of talking in my sleep, and sometimes I even sleepwalk. As a kid, it was really bad: I would often wake up standing on my bed shouting and punching the air, and I once peed in the corner of my sister's bedroom thinking it was the bathroom. On that long flight, as everyone slept, the cabin lights low, I was attacked with another bout of night terrors. All of a sudden, I jumped out of my seat, neck pillow dangling, eye mask covering one eye, looking like a pirate, and started yelling, "Who's flying this plane, we're going down, who's flying the plane?!" Amanda quickly tackled me and pulled me back into the seat. I'd woken the whole plane up, and she apologized to everyone and explained that I was sleep-talking and that everything was fine.

It was two in the morning when we touched down in Mumbai. Outside the air was thick and humid and smelled of cumin, cardamom, and petrol. We moved through the swarm of human beings, looking for a taxi. A crowd of mostly men, smoking bidis and drinking chai, stood next to their rickshaws. The sound of blaring horns and the bells of indifferent cows bobbing through the traffic created a cacophony of dense noise. It was music to my ears. I remembered what Pietro told me in the small church outside of Rome: the universe is serenading itself, and we are all a part of the orchestra.

We spotted an old black-and-yellow taxi with a statue of Ganesh on the dashboard. "A good omen," I said to Amanda. We threw our backpacks in the trunk and slid into the back seat. The driver was a very kind old man with a long beard and gentle eyes. When I introduced myself he turned to face us, and in the most joyful voice he said, "Welcome to India, brother. My name is Ganesh!" I looked at Amanda and smiled.

We had booked our first night's stay at a hotel we found on the Internet. When we arrived, the place was a lot shabbier than the pictures on their website. When the clerk turned the lights on in the hallway to take us to our room, we saw several mice scatter and run into the shadows. "Another good omen!" said Amanda, laughing, because Ganesh, the elephant god of fortunate blessings, is known for riding on a mouse.

We were delirious. Our room was so dirty that we slept in our clothes, but we were happy—happy to be horizontal after the long flight, happy to be in India, and happy to be together. When morning came a few hours later we shared a granola bar that we had brought from home and started to plan our first adventure. We wanted to start our trip in the most auspicious way possible, so we decided to visit the famous temple devoted to Lakshmi, the goddess of wealth and beauty. Before we checked out of our grungy hotel, I shaved off all my hair in the bathroom sink to symbolically let go of the past and prepare for this sacred journey.

The Lakshmi temple in Mumbai stood on the edge of the city overlooking the Arabian Sea. The road leading to the temple was lined with stalls selling flowers, incense, and sweets. We made our purchases, removed our shoes, and then stood in line to make our offerings to the goddess. As we approached the altar, the priest at the temple invited us to light several sticks of incense. He chanted mantras as he marked our foreheads with crimson-red powder and tied brightly colored cotton threads around our wrists. We bowed our heads to receive the blessings.

Outside the temple, we walked down the stairs and then out onto the slippery black rocks to stand at the edge of the ocean. Placing a lotus flower into the water, Amanda and I shared our own personal prayer. *May this journey bring us closer together and deepen our understanding of yoga. May we be blessed, may we be safe, and may we be guided by Grace.*

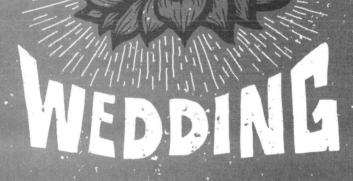

Krishna's WEDDING

22

KRISHNA'S WEDDING

WE DIDN'T LINGER IN MUMBAI LONG BUT HEADED south to Chennai, where we had been invited to attend the wedding of our friend Krishna, who we knew from the yoga studio back home. Krishna, like many young Indian men with an engineering degree, had found work in San Francisco during the tech boom. He was from a traditional Brahmin family, and he'd only met his fiancée through emails. It was an arranged marriage. The idea of my parents picking out my life partner was a hard concept to wrap my head around. Krishna was kind, but also painfully shy, so I imagine it must have been helpful for him to have his family's support.

When we arrived we were greeted with a great deal of fanfare. We were the only Westerners to attend the wedding, and Krishna's family was thrilled that we made it all the way from California. The day before the ceremony, a group of Krishna's aunties took us shopping in the local village to help us buy proper clothes for the wedding. They helped Amanda pick out a beautiful gold-and-white sari. The tailor was able to stitch her a custom top in just a few hours while I picked out my outfit, a traditional wheat-colored men's kurta, or long collarless shirt, worn over a pair of loose-fitting pajama pants.

When we emerged from the hotel room in our new clothes, we were completely transformed. The aunties had helped Amanda to wrap her sari and had pushed tight glass bangles over her wrists. They giggled as they helped her dress, like they were playing with a life-size doll. When they were done, they strung a garland of jasmine flowers in her hair and placed a jeweled *bindi* in the center of her forehead. She looked like a princess.

We made our way to the banquet hall, where we were given seats of honor next to Krishna's ninety-year-old grandfather, who welcomed us with a warm smile. His voice was soft and kind, and his old eyes were filled with a deep wisdom. He told me about the time he met Mahatma Gandhi, and his experience during the independence movement.

The marble floor of the wedding hall was cool on my bare feet. Vedic priests wrapped in simple clean white cotton rang brass bells and blew into conch shells, blessing the space, while streams of incense smoke curled in the air. Krishna and his soon-to-be wife sat on a royal throne. The dais was an ornately carved stage made of metal, with plush red velvet cushions. The bride was adorned with heavy jewels falling from her ears, fore-head, and neck. Rows of gold bangles wrapped around her arms, and the edges of her eyelids were lined with black kohl. She looked like a queen at a coronation.

The ceremony was long and elaborate. The priests continued to feed the fire with fragrant herbs, oil, and ghee as they chanted mantras. The flames rose up to catch the offerings. Every so often Krishna's grandfather would lean over and explain to us what was happening.

There was a profound moment when the bride's father symbolically gave his daughter away. He held his grown daughter on his knee one last time and then gave her to her husband. Then a priest tied a sacred thread to bind husband and wife together. There was so much emotion in the bride's face: fear, joy, and sadness all mixed together. I could only imagine what she was feeling in that moment. We knew that after the wedding she would be leaving her family for real and going with her new husband, a man she barely knew, to America.

After they were tied together, Krishna and his wife took seven sacred steps around the fire. Each step was a vow and symbolized a new layer of their commitment to one another. I imagined what it would be like to take those same steps with Amanda. On the seventh and last step, Krishna's grandfather leaned over to us and whispered, "This is where they promise, above all else, to remain friends."

At the end of the ceremony the couple was showered with rice and flower petals. Krishna's grandfather threw some at the couple on the stage and then turned to us, beaming through his kind and ancient face, and threw a handful of flowers over our heads. "There's a saying in India: weddings are arranged in heaven and celebrated on earth."

It was a great honor to be there for Krishna, and to meet his family. As the band played triumphant music and everyone took pictures, I thought about the significance of commitment in relationships. After the ceremony I asked Krishna's grandfather if he could tell me more about the meaning of the seven steps. This is what I remember:

The first step is to nourish each other, the second step is to grow strong together, the third step is to be successful, the fourth step is to share our joys and sorrows, the fifth step is to take care of our family, the sixth step is to stay together, and the seventh step is to be friends in this world and the next.

The wedding reminded me how lucky I was to be with Amanda. I had found someone to share the path with, and now that we were together, I never wanted to leave her side.

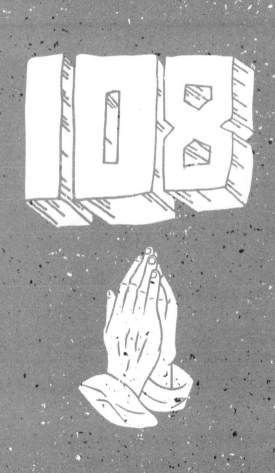

23

108

FTER THE WEDDING WE THANKED KRISHNA AND his family and continued on our journey. We had heard about a saint who was famous for his ability to manifest objects out of thin air. I was intrigued, and decided this was something I wanted to see for myself. The saint's ashram was in Karnataka, and I convinced Amanda we should go there on the way to Mysore. When we arrived we saw a massive white building, with beautiful statues guarding the door. Across the street was an open-air bazaar teeming with activity. As my eyes wandered I could see all the stalls filled with every kind of plastic souvenir you could imagine. The image of the saint was on everything, from calendars and huge laminated photos to coffee mugs, limited-edition coins, key chains, and even snow globes.

After speaking to some of the locals, Amanda and I found a place to stay in the home of a Muslim family just fifteen minutes' walking distance from the ashram. The family was renting out their rooms to traveling devotees, and the place was perfect.

We stayed upstairs in a room that looked like the inside of a jewelry box. The ceiling was painted light blue, and the walls were a creamy pink, framed with dark cherrywood molding. The ceiling fan whipped cool air into the room, and as soon as we walked in I collapsed onto the gold polyester sheets that covered the bed. That night I slept all the way through into the morning. No sleepwalking or sleep-talking, just deep, satisfying rest that lasted till dawn. When I woke up I shot out of bed, anxious to go find out how and when we could meet the saint.

Later that day, we wandered back to the spiritual marketplace, where we met some of the saint's followers who traveled from around the world to be with their guru. The devotees were so excited to share their stories about the saint's great acts of charity and all the miracles he had performed. One woman was adamant that he wasn't just a saint but the one and only living avatar of God.

Walking around the ashram grounds, we met a young Indian man named Prakash. Prakash was a college student and was visiting the ashram during his break. I asked Prakash what his name meant. He smiled. "It means 'sunlight' or 'bright light,'" he said. As we sat together in the sun-drenched courtyard of the ashram, Prakash noticed the row of *rudraksha* beads hanging from my neck. "Those are very good for protection," he said. "Do you practice chanting mantras?"

"I do," I replied, "but not so much with the beads. I usually just repeat them in my head."

"That is very good. If you like I can also show you how to use the beads to practice your mantras."

Prakash pulled his own necklace, or *mala*, from his pocket. "Use your right hand only. The left hand is used to clean yourself in the latrine, and shouldn't touch the *mala*. Extend your right pointer figure like this," he continued, showing me. "The pointer finger should never touch the *mala*, either. The pointer finger represents the ego, the small self which in Sanskrit is called *ahamkara*. Hold the *mala* with your thumb and ring finger. The thumb represents God: it's very hard to use your hand without a thumb; like that, everything becomes impossible without the support of the Creator." It reminded me of a soda we'd seen all over India, a bottle with the picture of a thumbs-up on it. "Is that why the most popular soda in India is Thums Up?" I joked. "Maybe you are right!" Prakash said, laughing.

"Use your thumb and second finger to pass the beads," he instructed. I was starting to get the hang of it; it was like using chopsticks for the first time. "Perfect," he said. "Just like that. Now, there's one thing you should know. There are one hundred and eight beads on this *mala*. You see, there are one hundred and eight subtle doors in the heart; each time you chant your mantra you are opening one of those doors. Once all of them are open, my friend, then you will experience an exalted state of ecstasy."

"Now, the last thing you must remember," Prakash continued, "is when you come to the final bead, the one that sticks out, higher than the rest, this is the guru bead; you must never cross it." "Why?" I asked. Prakash paused, took a deep breath, and then continued, "The guru is above all else, and I don't mean just the human being we call guru or teacher, but Guru with a capital G. That Guru is the supreme principal that inhabits every being in the form of intuition, the inner knowing and feeling that tells us whether or not something is true.

"There are human gurus who develop their *siddhis,* or spiritual powers. They can see above and beyond our mundane reality, and through all the superficialities of this world, but they, like us, are also imperfect beings working through their own karma. The bigger Guru, the eternal one behind all these teachers, is perfect beyond measure. God is the true Guru and the source of all the great teachings.

"So once you come to that bead," Prakash warned, instead of crossing it, "spin the *mala* with your thumb and middle finger and begin again. That way we stay humble and are reminded that everything begins and ends with the Divine."

Amanda and I thanked Prakash. I was amazed to have met someone so young who was full of so much knowledge. "And remember," Prakash said as we were leaving, "no matter what happens, keep practicing."

MYSTICS
Magicians
&
MADMEN

24

MYSTICS, MAGICIANS, AND MADMEN

HERE IS AN ANCIENT TRADITION IN INDIA CALLED *darshan,* which means "having the auspicious sight of a deity or holy person." It's like a mirror; it allows us to see and to be seen. The ashram held huge public programs where thousands would gather to meditate, chant, and wait for the appearance of the holy saint so they could experience *darshan.* Many devotees came to the program with handwritten letters requesting guidance from their guru. If your letter was chosen, you would get a private audience, where you could ask him questions and maybe even receive a special blessing. Word on the street was that sometimes in these private sessions the guru would manifest magical objects, including jewelry. When I heard that, I tore a blank page out of my sketchbook and began composing my letter to the saint.

Dear Holy Sir,

I am so grateful for the opportunity to be in your presence. I have traveled all the way from America to learn about yoga and would appreciate any guidance you could offer to a young student on the path.

The next morning I sat poised in the crowded field of the ashram with my letter, waiting with the rest of the eager devotees for the living saint to arrive. The audience was split into two sections: men sat on the right, and women sat on the left. My fingers were crossed in hopes he would see me so that I could be picked for a private audience. When he finally appeared, his presence dazzled the crowd. He wore long, flowing orange robes, and when he waved his hands, his body language and soft smile seemed to exude a divine energy. After the first day and no sign of him taking my letter, I thought to myself, *The destined date must be tomorrow.*

The next day I showed up even earlier, dressed in all white. Together with the huge crowd, we chanted and meditated. As the saint made his rounds, he didn't even come close to the area where I was sitting. After all was said and done, I looked down at my letter—still nothing. I hadn't given up hope, though. Maybe he was testing my resolve. *Tomorrow for sure,* I thought. *That's when it's going to happen.*

Several days passed, and still no recognition from the saint. It was our last day before we were scheduled to leave for Mysore. We went to the ashram one last time. I was still holding on to the hope that the saint was going to take my letter. I waited nervously, holding the folded piece of paper like a gambling addict clings to a lotto ticket. As the music grew I started chanting louder and louder, until I was the loudest voice in the crowd. I was gathering and mustering my energy, trying to make my aura bigger, all in the hopes of being seen and acknowledged by the enlightened one.

In the midst of my guru madness, I'd also convinced myself that not only was I going to get picked to have a private audience but that he was going to manifest a diamond wedding ring so I could propose to Amanda.

As the saint walked onto the stage I could feel his magnetism. *Finally,* I thought, *I'm going to be with the saint and he's going to perform his miracle for me.* As he glided across the stage, the music and the chanting swelled. A great wave of excitement swept the crowd.

The saint sat on his throne-like chair, like a spiritual rock star. I felt my attachment and desire growing to a fever pitch. *I have to give him this letter,* I thought. After thirty more minutes of chanting, he stood up and began to glide through the audience, selecting letters and offering blessings. *This is it,* I thought. *He's going to take my letter for sure and invite me back for an interview behind the curtains of the stage.*

I watched with unbroken concentration as he floated through the crowd. I was drunk with anticipation. My mantra morphed into *Pick me, pick me, pick me.* When I couldn't take it anymore, I stood up and began climbing over everyone in my row with the desperation of a drowning person trying to get to a lifeboat. The guru was just a few yards away. I held my letter with my outstretched hand, emphatically waiving it.

His back was to me, and all I needed was for him to turn around. As the saint pivoted to face me, *BOOM!* I was tackled by the Indian security guards. It was a dog pile, and I was at the bottom. As I looked up through the bodies of the security guards and saw the orange robe floating away, I held my spiritual letter and continued shaking it in the air.

I was quickly escorted out of the ashram. Amanda, having seen the whole drama unfold from the women's side of the field, met me at the entrance and just shook her head. I was so embarrassed.

I began my long walk of shame back to our rented room. While walking with my head hung low, a young boy appeared out of nowhere. "You're in luck," he said. "Right this way for a very special once-in-a-lifetime astrology reading." I was feeling ungrounded and hungry to know whether or not the guru was ever going to acknowledge me. I convinced Amanda that we should follow the boy and learn what the astrologer might have to say.

The boy led us through a series of back alleyways to a ramshackle house. In the back corner of the yard there was an old dilapidated shed. "Please, right this way," the boy whispered as he ushered us in. Two empty plastic lawn chairs sat in front of an old desk covered with piles of papers and dusty relics. Just behind the chairs there hung a framed photo of the saint behind a pane of cracked glass, and above the photo a single lightbulb was glowing.

The moment I sat down, I turned around to look at the image, and as I stared into the eyes of the saint, the light bulb flickered and burned out. Amanda looked at me and said, "I have a strange feeling about this place. Maybe we should go." Just then an older man appeared with a stack of books under his arm. He didn't speak much English, so the young boy translated for him. Together they explained the menu of prices, pitching different astrological services. "Just a basic reading is good," I said.

We gave him the details of our births. As the astrologer crunched his numbers, scribbling notes on a folded piece of paper, his eyes would look up into mine; then his head would drop again as he scribbled more chicken scratch on the page. He opened a drawer and pulled out a small bag of what looked like animal bones. He collected them in his left palm, shook them, and then rolled the bones like dice.

As he spoke the young boy translated. "You will become great devotees of the saint, and visit at least seven more times. On your third visit you will get a private audience. By then you will be married and have two children." The tone of the old man's voice changed as he went on. "At some point in your life you were walking down a dark path and came across black magic. It wasn't yours, but you became involved in it, and now it has affected your journey. Fortunately, you found me, and for an extra fee, a mere three hundred U.S. dollars, we can organize a very sacred ceremony with our community of priests to remove this black magic from your life."

It became clear to me that the only black magic I needed to remove was the one that was being presented to me at that table. "No thank you, I'm not going to pay any extra. Please just finish." The encounter with the backdoor astrologer took a turn for the worse as he began to read Amanda's chart, giving her the date of her death, and then soliciting for more fees and more ceremonies.

The information shook me out of my trance, shattering the spell I was under. Amanda had a look of dread in her face, and seeing her like that quickly sobered me up. "That's enough," I said.

In that moment I realized what a fool I had been. I'd let my desire and attachment get the best of me. In my hunger to be noticed and to feel special, I'd completely lost track of what was important, what was real. I'd let myself become seduced by the hype machine surrounding the saint, and worst of all I had led Amanda into a terrible situation with this charlatan astrologer.

We left quickly and hurried back to the safety of our hotel room. As we packed up our things and got ready to leave, I remembered the words of Prakash, who had taught me how to use my *mala*. He had been trying to teach me about discernment and how to determine whether something was true or false. I was just beginning to understand this deep teaching, yet some part of me knew then that if I was going to navigate this spiritual journey I would have to get better at listening to my own inner guide.

25

FROM DARKNESS TO LIGHT

I HUNG FROM THE SIDE OF THE TRAIN LOOKING OUT across the endless rice fields as they rushed by. The dense green hills in the distance were lined with rows of palm trees, and I could see young men scaling them, ascending the long narrow trunks, knocking coconuts down from above. The sound of the Beastie Boys' *Check Your Head* filled my headphones, reminding me of home, as we made our way to Mysore, the city of yoga.

When we arrived at the train station, we met a rickshaw driver named Shiva. Shiva had a long black beard, dark eyes, and a mischievous smile. He welcomed us, saying, *"Namaste,"* and as we threw our bags in the back, a familiar song filled my ears. His rickshaw was equipped with a sweet sound system. "Is that Bob Marley?" I asked. "Yes!" Shiva smiled. "'Buffalo Soldier,' that is my number-one favorite song," he said as he held his pointer finger up and waved it. "Do you like Bob Marley?" he asked. "Who doesn't?" I replied. "Well then," Shiva said, "let's turn it up!"

The sound of reggae music filled the air as Shiva wove his way through clusters of traffic. Inside of the rickshaw Amanda and I smiled at each other. "I can't believe we made it to Mysore," she said. We gazed out into the crowded streets, trying to take it all in. Hindu temples dotted the city with brightly colored spires, each tower decorated with ornately carved figures. Gods and goddesses like Ganesha and Lakshmi floated above us as we sped down the busy roads. The street art covering the walls was vibrant against the decay of the ancient buildings. Sacred images depicting divine characters, Om symbols, and mythic heroes were everywhere. I noticed that most of the signage and the lettering in the street was hand-painted. The bold script with its intricate details and punchy bright colors grabbed my attention. Everywhere I looked it seemed like India was covered in spiritual graffiti.

The city of Mysore was majestic. Shiva explained how it was built around a beautiful palace that lights up every Sunday night. The maharaja was a great man, he said. He helped to bring yoga out of the shadows during a time when it was looked down upon because of the British. Shiva took us by the palace so we could check it out. As we were driving past the massive archways, I noticed a towering hill off in the distance. I asked Shiva about it. "That, my friend, is Chamundi Hill. There are

1,008 steps that lead to a temple at the summit, which sits above the city like a spiritual crown. It's where the great goddess named Durga slayed the buffalo demon, Mahishasura. The city's name, Mysuru, or Mysore, comes from the name of the slain demon. This is the land of the victorious goddess."

When we arrived we met up with another young couple from San Francisco who were also there to study yoga. The four of us shared an unfurnished house. Amanda and I had intended to practice with Shri K. Pattabhi Jois, but when we arrived I realized there were different schools where I could study. Someone told me about another teacher, younger and less famous, named Yogacharya Venkatesh, who ran a center for yogic sciences with his wife and offered a full program that included *asana*, meditation, philosophy, chanting, and Sanskrit. The idea of getting a more well-rounded education from a teacher who spoke fluent English and was more accessible appealed to me. Amanda decided to study with Shri K. Pattabhi Jois, and I signed up to study with Acharya Venkatesh.

Acharya was in his early thirties. When I met him he was wearing a clean white button-down shirt and had a thick brown mustache. Acharya was very straightforward and to the point. He set out clear rules and regulations for practicing at his school. I was to be on time; no exceptions, or I would not be allowed to practice. There were no drop-ins; students had to commit to an extensive course and were expected to dress modestly. Both men and women were required to wear T-shirts at all times; no shirtless men, or women in sports bras. He liked us to keep our belongings contained and tidy, and all around the school there were hand-painted reminders—like "Do Not Scatter the Slippers," which hung over the bench where we left our shoes. The structure reminded me of my old group home, which was comforting.

Once I committed to the program, our study together was vigorous. He always pushed me to go deeper, and it wasn't just in the postures. "Yoga is about learning to bend the mind," he'd say. "The body is just a tool." He told me that many students would come to Mysore and be interested only in physical practice, and instead of advancing their yoga they would injure themselves from doing too much too fast. Acharya felt it was important to view yoga as more of a marathon and less of a sprint. He'd say things like, "It's better to walk every day for an hour than not do anything for six months and then try to run twenty miles in one day. It's not about more, more, more," he told me, "it's about a slow, steady, regular practice, gradually, over a long period of time. If you do too much right away you will burn out. You must remember this is a lifelong discipline: there are no shortcuts."

During my three months in Mysore, every day I'd wake up at 4 A.M. and ride a very heavy, rusty bicycle several miles through the city, pushing it uphill so I wouldn't be late. Meditation was always first. I'd take my seat on the concrete floor and sit until Acharya said it was time to practice postures. One morning Acharya placed a candle in front of me. He instructed me to stare at it without blinking and without moving. Before long, attracted by the light and my body heat, a swarm of hungry mosquitoes began hovering around my head as I tried to stay focused on the flame. I had to resist every urge to swat the mosquitoes and maintain my concentration. This practice was called *trataka* and was meant to purify my vision.

During another session, Acharya placed a big plastic red bucket and a tiny pink rubber hose in front of me. "What am I supposed to do, put a rubber hose up my nose?" I asked, jokingly. "Yes," he said, in an expressionless tone. He instructed me to thread the hose up my nose until it slid all the way down and the tip dangled at the back of my throat. The tricky part was reaching my fingers back without gagging. I almost threw up several times as I stuck my hand in my mouth. I connected the opposite ends of the hose and began flossing the tube through my nasal cavity. I have a big nose, so it wasn't that hard.

After I'd cleared my nostrils, Acharya handed me a neti pot—a small white porcelain cup that looks like a teapot filled with warm water and salt. Sticking the long spout up my nose, he instructed me to tip my head so it poured out the other side. My eyes crossed as I looked down, watching as the booger-filled waterfall spilled into the plastic red bucket. "Now I will show you *kapalabhati,* or skull-shining breath," he said. "Watch me first, and do exactly as I do." He demonstrated the fiery breath by exhaling rapidly through his nose while pressing his hands against his thighs. "Okay, now you do it," he instructed. *Kapalabhati—seems more like kapala-snotty,* I thought. I followed his instructions and began using my core muscles to push the air out through my nose, polishing the inside of my skull with my breath. Once we finished I took the deepest inhalation of my life. As oxygen flooded my entire system, my mind felt clear and bright.

"These are *kriyas* . . . or purification practices," Acharya explained. "They help to clear the nasal passage so you can breathe with more freedom. If you can steady the breath then you can steady the mind."

I learned invocations to the sun, chanting before each sun salutation. The practice was slow and careful, with a lot of attention on our alignment and breathing while we moved. As the weeks progressed, so did my studies. When I started, I was sitting for only ten minutes in meditation, but after a few months I was sitting for forty-five minutes. Meditation was starting to become easier, thanks to the *sattvic,* or pure food, that Acharya's family had been preparing for Amanda and me every day. A three-tiered stainless-steel tiffin box filled with vegetarian food and a fresh coconut became my reward after an intensive day of practice.

The part of the program I enjoyed the most was learning to chant in Sanskrit. Amanda would join me for these sessions after she was done practicing with Pattabhi Jois. We were taught by Acharya's wife, Hema, who was my age: only twenty-one. She had grown up in a spiritual family and started learning the Bhagavad Gita, one of the yoga tradition's most sacred texts, at age five. When she taught us verses, she didn't use a book but instead let it flow from her deep personal experience, providing us with a fresh and authentic translation every time. We sat and listened, and when it was time to sing together, Hema would teach us a few simple prayers. This is one of the beautiful chants we learned.

Om asatomā sadgamaya / tamasomā jyotir gamaya
mrityormāamritam gamaya / Om śhānti śhāntiḥ

From ignorance, lead me to truth;
From darkness, lead me to light;
From death, lead me to immortality
Om peace, peace, peace

This chant resonated with me deeply because it reminded me of my own journey, from violence and drugs and all the confusion I experienced when I was younger to the peace and discipline I was now experiencing thanks to yoga.

I am so grateful for the time I spent with Acharya Venkatesh and Hema. Seeing a husband and wife teaching yoga side by side in such a sincere and dedicated way created a very deep and profound impression in my mind that would stick with me long after Amanda and I returned to San Francisco.

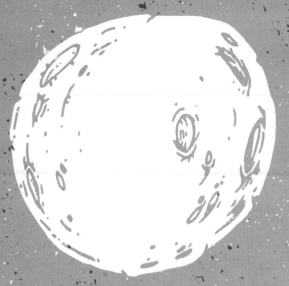

Visions

UNDER

THE FULL

MOON

26

VISIONS UNDER THE FULL MOON

A FTER COMPLETING OUR THREE MONTHS OF YOGA training in Mysore, Amanda and I decided on one last adventure before leaving India. We'd seen so much during our stay—we'd spent time volunteering at an orphanage for girls, visited the largest monolithic statue in the world, marched in a parade, met a bodybuilder named Mr. India, helped raise money for the earthquake victims in Gujarat, and even checked out an Indian water park, where women slid down the slides in their saris. There was only one thing left to do, and that was to fulfill my dream of seeing a tiger in the wild!

Together with a few of our yoga friends, we arranged to go on a jungle safari in the Rajiv Gandhi National Park. The nature reserve was seated deep in the forest of Karnataka. It was a sprawling landscape of teak, rosewood, and sandalwood trees—a refuge for Bengal tigers and several other rare species. There were sloths lounging in the trees, wild boars rustling in the bush, and four-horned antelopes and barking deer grazing in the fields. I saw striped hyenas, jungle bison, and majestic elephants all living in the jungle harmoniously.

We headed toward the main bungalow house. The man in charge greeted our crew of yogis and nature enthusiasts. We gathered in the main living room sipping fresh lime soda as Sahib, the man in charge, began telling us all about the wonders of the jungle and the magic that hid in her foliage. "The preserve is a refuge for wild tigers," he said, "and if you're lucky you'll have the *darshan* of one."

Tigers are revered in India, our guide said. Even the goddess Durga rides one as she heroically slays a demon who has taken over the world. Yogis revere animals and see them as teachers, he said. They are enlightened beings in disguise who impart great blessings and wisdom. The wisdom of the tiger reminds us to be calm and relaxed, conserving our energy so we can strike with full force when it's time to take action.

As the day fell into night, we settled in. The next morning we all climbed into a jeep, ready to explore the jungle. We drove to the edge of the water, where we took a boat ride across a beautiful glassy lake filled with blooming lotuses unfolding on all sides, opening to greet the sun. "What's that?" I asked, pointing to what looked like a log. Sahib pressed his binoculars to his face. "That, my boy, is a crocodile, and if you look down there right next to you, there is another one!" I jumped. I real-ized most of the logs were crocodiles; they were floating everywhere.

Once we got back to shore, I saw a tiny hint of or-ange in the distance. "Is that . . .?" I asked. "Yes, I be-lieve so," Sahib said in a hushed tone. "It is very rare to see one, and you are lucky even to have a small glimpse." After making friends with some wild elephants and watching the peacocks show off their colors, we made our way back to the bungalow. As the sun sank into the hills, the insects began their symphony.

It was a full-moon night, and Sahib told Amanda and me about a tree that hung over the lake that we could climb. At the top was an incredible tree house. We carefully climbed up the rope ladder, and once we made it to the platform, we sat together looking out across the lake as the moon reflected its light in the water below. We decided to meditate.

As I quieted down, I became completely absorbed in the sounds of the jungle. The air was the same tempera-ture as my body. I felt my shoulders soften, sliding down my back as my spine grew longer. As my mind turned inward, I saw a glimmer of light in the center of my body. It started to spread, shining in my bones and blood, and I could feel it move in and out with my breath. I saw my glowing body sitting next to Amanda high up in the tree house, with the lake of lotuses below us and the full moon overhead. As my vision expanded, it pulled out to reveal the expanse of the entire jungle:

I could see all the animals, including the elephants and Bengal tigers. Soon, I could see all of South India. Like the power of ten, my mind pulled out even more, revealing the Eastern Hemisphere covered in darkness as the sun shone against the opposite side of the earth. Pulling back even more, I saw the earth hanging like an earring in the sky, surrounded by billions of stars swirling in space, infinite clusters of galaxies. Everything became luminous. I felt that all of it was inside me. It was like I had an enormous cosmic body, and in my vision I saw Amanda sitting beside me in her own equally radiant cosmic body.

After an hour of sitting, my eyelids were heavy. I slowly peeled them open and saw Amanda opening hers at the same time. "You're never going to guess what I just saw," Amanda said. My eyes were still adjusting to the moonlight; everything was soft and a little blurry. As Amanda began to share her vision, my mouth slowly opened. I listened to her recount her meditation, and by the time she was finished, my jaw was on the floor.

"Why are you looking at me like that?" she asked.

"That's exactly what I saw, too!" We had experienced rhyming meditations.

Later on, after we had climbed down out of the treehouse and were back in our bungalow, we were still in awe of what had happened. Did we have some kind of mind-meld up there? What was the significance of the vision? We decided to write down our experience, and as we did, our rhyming meditation began to reveal its message to us. What came through was a mission statement for why we were together. The vision solidified what we had known since the beginning: our life together would be rooted in yoga.

As we prepared to go home, I thought about all that I had learned in India. My time in Mysore taught me discipline and that there are no shortcuts on this path. We have to do the work in order to experience all the blessings yoga has to offer. Being with the holy saint taught me discernment and how to trust my intuition and not give my power away. Krishna's wedding had taught me the power of devotion and that sometimes you need to surrender and trust in order to experience love. Discipline. Discernment. Devotion. As I contemplated these words, I began to see that they were the three keys to the door of yoga. The first key, discipline, the physical practice, unlocks the body. The second key, discernment, unlocks the mind to reveal what is true. And the third key, devotion, unlocks the heart.

DOORWAY TO

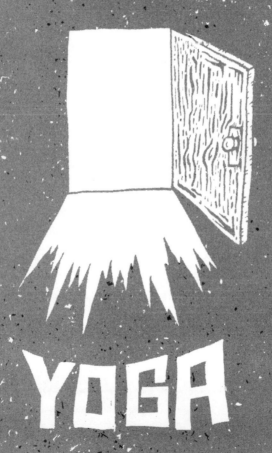

YOGA

27

DOORWAY TO YOGA

A FTER RETURNING FROM INDIA, AMANDA AND I DE-cided it was time to move in together. Our rhyming visions in the tree house were still echoing in both of our minds.

When we went to visit my dad at the store, I noticed there was a brand-new, bright red door on the side of the barn. The door had not been there before we left for India. I asked my dad about it. "It leads to yoga," he said with a smile. I was stunned. Before, we had to enter the yoga space through an old dark and dirty storeroom; the space was tucked so far in the back, no one even knew it was there. It was like an underground secret yoga cave.

Now there was a big bright red door, and handmade stairs that welcomed people into the space. I walked up the stairs and opened the door. There was the room where I first practiced yoga. It was as beautiful as ever. The wood floors seemed to be glowing. The smell of incense and fresh flowers flooded my senses, reminding me of India.

"What do you think?" my dad asked. "Feels like home," I said. "I'm a little confused, though. I thought this was your personal space for you and your friends to practice in."

"Well," my dad said, "now that you're back from India, I was thinking that maybe you and Amanda could start teaching classes." Larry had told me that yoga would open doors I never knew existed. It was decided there and then that we would open our own yoga studio.

Amanda and I found a place to live in a little town just north of my dad's store. Our place was small, cheap, and not very well insulated. When it rained, there were leaks all over the place. It was pretty bare-bones, but we were happy to have our first home together.

Starting our yoga studio was like a having a new baby. It involved a huge learning curve and required almost constant care. While the studio was growing, we both worked two other jobs to help pay our bills. Amanda worked two days a week for her sister's dog hotel and did freelance graphic design. I worked part-time loading and delivering hay at my dad's store and also worked at the local pizzeria.

We made some flyers and put them up around town. We designed everything ourselves, from the signs to the schedules, and Amanda built the website. When the day came to open the doors to the public, we drew straws, and I taught the first class. I was so nervous. I'd taught in the city under Larry's guidance, but now it was my own studio, and I felt incredibly self-conscious and filled with doubt. Five people showed up to that first class, and two of them were Amanda and my dad.

Halfway through the class, my nerves overcame me so much that I actually walked into the closet where we stored our yoga props behind a curtain, to hide. I took a few breaths and then poked my head out and asked if people still liked me and if they wanted to continue the class. Amanda and I went on to teach all the classes for the first seven years, and a lot of incredible things happened during that time. We taught seventeen classes a week, 364 days a year, every day except Christmas. Whenever something needed to be fixed or taken care of, we figured it out.

Not only were we the only teachers, we also were the manager, accountant, janitor, gardener, marketing team, etc. If a mouse died under the studio, I'd suit up, grab my flashlight, and crawl under the building. It wasn't glamorous, but it was ours and we loved it.

It took a long time to build up a student base. We taught a lot of classes with just one or two people in them. Once, when we were two years in, Amanda called me, excited, to tell me that she had twelve students in a 6 P.M. class! Gradually, though, word spread and more students continued to come, so much so that about five years in we needed to expand the room because we were at capacity. Amanda's dad helped us make the investment in remodeling, and we added a boutique and French doors leading out to a small Zen garden. My uncle Gilbert came out and helped us create a pond for the garden. It was with a lot of pride and feeling of satisfaction that we did so much at our studio. It was truly a labor of love.

One day when I was teaching a morning class, all the locals showed up and one by one unrolled their mats and set up for practice. It was an average day, around twenty students. I walked in, greeted everyone, and off we went. As we moved through our warm-ups, flowing through the sun-salutation sequence, I pulled the curtains open and let the sunlight pour in. "Now let's strengthen our balance and coordination. Tree posture," I called out. "Lift your left leg, feel the power of the right leg." As the room stood together in tree pose, like a forest of yogis, I noticed an odd smell.

Then I saw a bright flash of light. There, in the corner, one of the students was standing in tree pose with her hair on fire. She had been standing near the altar on the wall, and a small tea light candle had ignited the top layer of her frizzy hair. Somehow she hadn't noticed it yet, and she stood peacefully as a bright orange flame wrapped around her head like a halo. There was a collective gasp as the room began to notice. I grabbed a yoga blanket, ran to the corner, and put out the fire. "OK, everybody, second side," I said, and to the class's credit they switched legs and kept breathing, without skipping a beat.

The student was a local lady, and one of the sweetest women in town. She confided in me afterward that she'd been telling herself all week, "I've been running around like my hair is on fire." The moment she said that my eyes got big. *Life is so bizarre,* I thought. *You can't make this stuff up.* Our thoughts are so powerful. I realized in that moment that everything we think, do, and say has the power to affect our reality. I remembered Larry's words: "We're stronger than we think we are."

So many other incredible things happened, some visible, some invisible. Teaching yoga in a small town, we really got to know our students, and a lot of them came to class to deal with major life transitions like recovering from a miscarriage, divorce, death of a family member, or cancer. They also came to the studio to celebrate their birthdays, their wedding days, and to meet and connect with friends. Just as Amanda and I had, some people met at our studio, fell in love, and got married. What developed over the years at the studio was a real sense of family and community. It's one of the things I'm most proud of.

One student came to me in his eighties; Stormin' Norman was the nickname I gave him. Norman was a transplant from New York City, a graduate of Juilliard, and he was a conductor in the Santa Cruz Symphony. Norman couldn't have been taller than five feet; his thick New York accent punctuated his far-left politics; and whenever I saw him he was always in the process of traveling the world or composing new music. Norman and I became close. He'd get us tickets to the symphony, join us for dinner at our house, and always be a source of good fun and laughter. He was a good friend.

Norman practiced with us into his late eighties, all the way up to the time he passed away. He never married or had children of his own, so it was his nephew who asked me to preside over his funeral rites. I felt it was a great honor that his family asked me to do that. On that beautiful Sunday, a small group of us gathered at the edge of the creek. I held the ashes of my friend in my hand. As a gentle breeze blew across the wetlands, I opened my palm and let the wind sweep Norman's remains into the creek that spills into the bay and opens into the ocean.

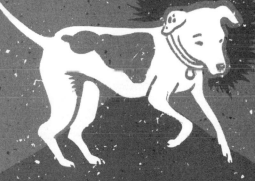

ENTER THE

MAHATMA

28

ENTER THE MAHATMA

NOT ALL MY TEACHERS WERE HUMANS. AMANDA was working a couple of days a week with her sister at her dog hotel, Citizen Canine, in Oakland. When they got busy, I would help out, too, shoveling huge piles of gravel in the yard and scooping more dog poop than I'd like to remember. It was a fun job, though. I enjoyed seeing all the different kinds of dogs and hearing the crazy stories about their owners. One dog was dropped off with the specific order that she must watch *Oprah* every day; another dog, we were told, could drink water only from a crystal glass. I loved all the dogs, and to this day I can still remember some of the regular visitors like Handsome Bob the basset hound—and Lucy the Maltese, who needed to be watched very closely in the yard because she liked to eat other dogs' poo.

Because Citizen Canine was next door to the SPCA, people dropped stray dogs off at their doorstep all the time. Even though Amanda's sister, Tina, was running a for-profit hotel, she had a big heart, and worked with local dog-rescue organizations to help foster and find homes for strays. That's how I met The Mo. When I first met him, he was in bad shape. A stray pit-bull mix from the streets of Oakland, he was scared, and most likely had been abused. The people who found Mo originally named him Dash because they saw him running in and out of traffic.

All the rooms were full, so Tina let Mo live in the men's room. The first time I met Mo, he barked liked crazy. I jumped back, not knowing that making direct eye contact with dogs is a sign of aggression. But even as he barked and growled, the hair on the back of his neck standing up—even underneath all that fear and anxiety, I felt a deep connection with him.

He was a mutt, but his prominent jawline and beautiful face showed that he was mostly a pit bull. He was taller and leaner than most pits, though. One of our friends who worked for a vet said that he was probably mixed with a hound and bred to be bait dog. Bait dogs are raised for one purpose: dying in dogfights. Mo was a survivor. He was good with women but terrified of men. I realized very quickly that he wanted nothing to do with me.

Fear lives in the mind, not in the soul, and even though I couldn't get near him, somehow I knew Mo was my soul friend. He was my dog, and I was his boy.

How can I explain that feeling, that deep knowing? It's that same knowing I felt when I first saw Amanda. Some things bypass the mind and go straight to the heart.

That first night after meeting Mo, I dreamt of him. In my dreams he was smiling, with his big, white-and-tan, beautiful face. He was like a deer, bouncing through fields of grass, blades bending beneath his paws, as he flew through the endless rolling hills in my mind. For the next few weeks all I could think about was Mo. Any excuse to go see him. Shovel dog shit? I thought you'd never ask. I made so many trips across the Bay Bridge just to be close to him.

Finally I told Amanda I couldn't live without him. I didn't care how hurt he was; we needed to bring him home. Amanda agreed, and the next day we drove to Oakland to adopt our boy.

I opened the door to the men's room where Mo was nesting. He looked up, but this time he didn't growl; he was happy to see me. We'd earned each other's trust after several months of me visiting and bringing him treats. Often I'd be coming from the ashram where I was meditating, so my energy was peaceful and calm. He knew my smell.

When we opened our yoga studio, we would bring Mo to class with us. Having a traumatized pit bull barking at your students as they enter the studio is not the best way to initiate a relaxing yoga experience. Fortunately, the students in our tiny northern Californian town were supercool and understanding.

Mo liked the ladies, but he would often freak out when a tall man came to yoga. I would do my best to console Mo, and I set up a bagel bed and blanket for him in the corner next to the heater. Once the class began, he would curl up and watch from the sidelines. As we pressed our palms together and began chanting Om, his ears would perk up, and he even joined in a few times with a purring howl.

After a few rounds of sun salutations, everyone would start sweating and dropping into the rhythm of their practice. Meanwhile, Mo would be melting in front of the heater. He'd roll over on his back, stretch his paws, and unroll his tongue as he yawned. As we flowed through our practice, he'd even join in with an occasional upward-facing dog and downward-facing dog. After the students moved through several rounds of heart-opening back bends and finishing postures, the class would dissolve into *shavasana.*

Every time without fail, during the final resting pose, Mo would climb out of his bagel bed and curl up between the legs of the same guy he had barked at at the beginning of class. He would snug himself in, rest his big pit-bull head on the guy's leg, and let out a sigh of contentment. It amazed me every time. That phenomenon happened for years—so many times in fact that Amanda and I used to say to the guys, "Don't worry, if he's barking at you now, he'll be your best friend in *shavasana.*"

Mo was short for Mahatma, which means "great soul" in Sanskrit, and the more yoga he was exposed to, the more he was slowly becoming his namesake. I named him that because on some level I knew there was a great spiritual being underneath all those *samskaras,* or mental scars. Over time, his heart unfolded, and without warning Mo, the traumatized pit bull, became a peaceful, enlightened yoga dog.

After being in the room for over ten thousand hours of yoga classes, seeing people enter in a state of stress, hurry, and worry and then be transformed, becoming more calm and steady through yoga, Mo learned to trust humans again.

After sixteen beautiful years of friendship, it was time to say good-bye. Mo had escaped several near-death experiences, but eventually age caught up with him. In the end he was diagnosed with lymphoma. On the day he was to be put down, Amanda and I held his furry body close. Our local vet, a woman who had cared for The Mo his whole life, came to our house. She made several attempts to euthanize him by injecting into his legs, but his veins were too swollen from his illness. Finally she apologized and said she would have to inject straight into his heart. Holding him in my arms, I watched as the needle pierced his chest. I braced myself for the pain of watching him go. But the moment I felt his body soften and his heartbeat still, instead of overwhelming loss, I felt my heart flood with overwhelming love and gratitude.

How lucky I was to have been able to live with and share such an intimate bond with this great and noble being. Mo became one of my greatest teachers. What was one of the hardest days of my life was also the most profoundly beautiful.

He taught me that death does not mean the end of a relationship, but a deepening of the love shared. He showed me that anyone can heal and turn their life around and that with enough love and patience there's hope for us all.

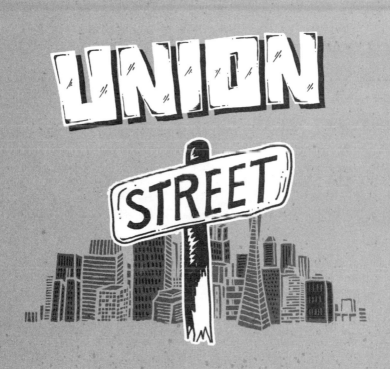

29

UNION STREET

HAD PROPOSED TO AMANDA BEFORE WE LEFT FOR India. We'd known each other for almost a year by then. When I got down on my knee and asked the question, she said yes, which was pretty amazing, considering I had no money, no job, and no car, was living with my dad, and had proposed to her using a ring I got out of a gum-ball machine. The ring was big, bright blue, and plastic; it had a sensor inside it, so that when I put it on her finger, it lit up.

My love for Amanda brought out the best in me. She made me to want to be a better person, a better man. When I met her I was young and didn't have much to offer, but I knew I wanted to give her the world, make her happy, be a great husband for her. The only problem was that I didn't really know how to do it. When I looked around, I didn't have many good role models. Most of the people I knew were either too afraid of getting hurt to even be in a relationship, single and sexually reckless, lying and cheating, or married and disgruntled, treating their spouses with thinly veiled animosity.

I wanted to experience something different, something better. When I shared with Larry that Amanda and I were engaged, he beamed with joy. He was so proud that we met through him. "If you're serious about making it work," he told me, "there's only one person you need to go see." "Who?" I asked. Larry smiled. "She's the oracle, the one who helped me find my way when I was first getting established. Her name is Dorothy Divack, and she lives on Union Street."

The first time I met Dorothy it was like meeting an African queen: her presence was regal and divine. She was not a yoga teacher in the way I was used to. Her lessons didn't involve getting on a mat and doing poses; instead she taught me how to integrate and embody the teachings of yoga. Dorothy herself was a master of her own mind, and because of her own clarity, she was able to see right through any spiritual bypass bullshit that I came up with. In those first years of working together she helped me navigate through my mental entanglements. She taught me how to be responsible for my thoughts, my words, and my actions. In some ways, it was the deepest version of yoga that I had ever practiced.

Her office was called the Center of Excellence, and she called the space where we met the Living Room of Consciousness. One day while I was sitting with her she asked me, "What's stopping you?" "Stopping me from what?" I asked. "What's stopping you from being fully present, fully committed?" I sat slumped in my chair. I felt the old layers of sleepiness and desire to go numb creep back in. "I'm going to invite you to sit up now and feel your feet on the ground," she said. Dorothy held space as I sat with the holding patterns I was harboring in the back of my mind. I did my best to stay with the feeling, the discomfort, instead of checking out, instead of distraction and instant gratification. Finally I felt it, the thing that was standing in the way. "It's a fear of failure," I said. "I don't think I'm good enough for Amanda."

"Keep going, take a few deep breaths," she said. "I'm worried we won't make it and that I'll lose the best thing that's ever happened to me," I told her. My mind clouded as all my insecurities rose to the surface. Dorothy looked me in the eyes; her gaze was penetrating. And that's when she gave me one of the most powerful teachings I'd ever received. *"Nothing real can be threatened. Nothing unreal exists. Only love is real."* It was a teaching from *A Course in Miracles,* a spiritual curriculum that Dorothy had studied and facilitated for over four decades.

Only love is real. Only love is real. Only love is real. I repeated it like a mantra. I could feel it slowly dissolving my fears, getting me below the chatter of my mind. The more I meditated on it, the more I could see how everything that had happened in the past had been driven by a desire for love. It bought up layers of pain and remorse. Remorse for all the times I'd stumbled, unskillfully trying to connect, using drugs and other destructive methods that gave me temporary relief but left a feeling of being even more disconnected afterward. Dorothy helped me move through it. I was starting to feel how love was underneath everything: it was the fiber and fabric of the universe, the underlying motivation; it encompassed not just my life, but everyone's. I could feel how we all share the same longing, the same desire to feel love and connection. It was deep. The teaching was helping me to become more compassionate toward myself and to the people in my life. The more I focused on the teaching, the more I found myself waking up to the power of love.

When the time came for Amanda and me to get married, three years after my proposal, Dorothy presided over the ceremony. We were married in our yoga studio, standing in the exact spot where I had first practiced yoga. Inspired by our time in India, we threaded rows of orange and red marigolds and hung them from the ceiling like curtains. At the end of the ceremony we invited all of our friends and family to chant Om with us.

My brother was my best man, and as a part of his best-man duties he lined up the music. The DJ he hired proceeded to play every classic wedding song you can imagine: "We Are Family" by Sister Sledge, "Celebration" by Kool and the Gang. When I requested some hip-hop, the DJ said, "Sure man, I've got the perfect track for you."

The squawk of a loud horn sent a jolt of energy through the party, and then the first words of the "Brass

Monkey" track dropped. It was the Beastie Boys. The heavy sound of the 808 drum slapped the speakers. A group of my friends started break-dancing in the middle of the dance floor. My friend Ross, who I'd studied yoga with in India, lifted up the statue of Hanuman, the monkey god, that lived on the altar of our yoga studio. "Look," he said, pointing excitedly, "Brass Monkey!"

A light bulb went off in my head. It was at that exact moment when two sides of myself came crashing together. Yoga and hip-hop.

Looking out, I could I see Amanda, Larry, Dorothy, and our entire families celebrating together. I thought to myself, *How could it possibly get better than this?*

BEASTIE

30

BEASTIE YOGI

HE DAY AFTER OUR WEDDING WE LEFT FOR OUR honeymoon in Hawaii. We stayed a couple of weeks on the island of Kauai. We loved everything about the North Shore, eating at the local hippie vegetarian restaurants, surfing at the beaches, and hiking the Napali Coast. We even found a sweet little yoga studio in the town of Hanalei that offered Mysore-style Ashtanga yoga. When we showed up for class, there were only two other students. One was the local baker, and the other was Mike D from the Beastie Boys.

During the practice, Mike D, the baker, Amanda, and I all helped each other out and offered each other assistance in some of the harder postures. It reminded me of my first experience practicing yoga in the barn with my dad and his carpenter friends. It was so relaxed and fun. Every once in a while I would pinch myself to make sure I wasn't dreaming. *Is this really my life right now?* I thought as I looked to my left and saw my beautiful wife and then to my right and saw one of my all-time hip-hop heroes, Mike D.

Sometimes after class, the four of us would get a juice from the stand across the street from the studio. Mike was so chill and friendly and down-to-earth. It was deeply inspiring to me to see that this guy could be both a hip-hop megastar and also a devoted yogi.

My encounter with Mike D in Hawaii relit my desire to make music and be an emcee. For the rest of our honeymoon I started writing lyrics with a vengeance. I filled three whole notebooks on that trip.

When I got home, I realized that the last few years of pursuing yoga had led me on an incredible journey. I had found myself, my wife, and my calling. Now it was time to find my creative outlet. I reached out to my brother, Adam, who was making a name for himself spinning records and promoting parties as DJ Amen. He knew a bunch of guys who were in the hip-hop scene but doing it in a more positive way than the kids I had hung out with when I was in school. These guys were not into battling or doing heavy drugs or getting arrested; they just wanted to be creative and have a way to express themselves.

One of the guys, Kel, an artist and fellow graffiti-head, knew about an old magnet factory called the Shop. The owners let people use the space to throw events for teens. Kel came up with the idea to have a regular hip-hop night there and invite all the local kids who were into DJing, rapping, breakdancing, and painting graffiti. He called it the Jam.

The Shop was covered from floor to ceiling with graffiti murals. Kel had organized a bunch of local graffiti writers to do fresh productions before the event. The night of the Jam, I was set to host with Kel, and be one of the main emcees alongside Emil, whom we called Emcee Sky Eye. Emil's family was from the Caribbean island of Martinique, and he could rap and sing in English and French, which I thought was so fresh.

As kids began to pour in, my cousin DJ Almighty and my brother DJ Amen warmed up the crowd by scratching records over live drum breaks. When it was time to jump on, Kel gave me the signal and Emil and I started pumping up the crowd. "If you came to get down and have fun tonight, let me hear you say . . . aaaallll-rrriiighht." The crowd responded, "Aaaalllllrrriiighht," as they started to press closer in toward the stage.

"Welcome to the Jam and I'm glad you're here. If you're ready for this, put your hands in the air." All the hands went up and started waving front to back. This crowd of sweaty teenagers was having fun, rocking their old-school Adidas tracksuits and striped tube socks. A circle began to form in the middle of the warehouse, and a crew of break-dancers, led by my friend Air Rock, began twisting and contorting to the beat, arms and legs flipped in all directions as the b-boys got down, energizing the dance floor. Behind me our other friend DJ Basta was throwing color across huge sheets of plywood, live-painting abstract graffiti-style words and symbols. Emil and I kept the party going with spontaneous freestyles and crowd-hyping chants. All the elements of hip-hop came together in one brilliant moment, the DJs scratching, the breakers breaking, the emcees rhyming and painters painting. It was a creative explosion of color and dynamic energy.

We kept the event drug, alcohol, and violence free, and because of that Kel was able to get sponsored by a local high school, which helped pay for the sound system. Every time, there were over a hundred kids that showed up to the Jam nights. It was a huge success, good times for everyone, and a great way for me to get back into emceeing.

I was a few years older than most of the kids there, and when I looked out onto the audience I was reminded of what life had been like for me as a teenager. I remembered how hard it was. I was so lucky I had found yoga when I did. Yoga had changed my life for the better, and now I had an opportunity to pay that forward and share what I had learned. I figured that most of the kids coming to the Shop had no idea what yoga was. If I could find a way to merge yoga philosophy with hip-hop, I just might be able to translate it into a language these kids could understand.

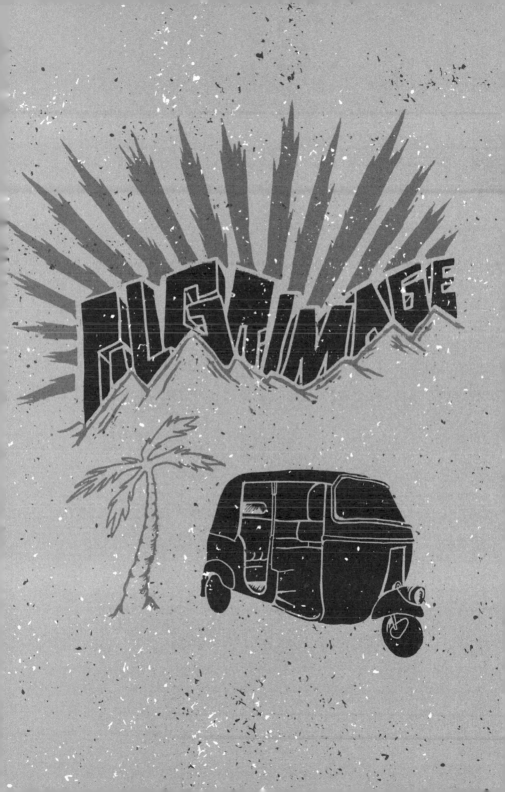

31

PILGRIMAGE

FTER A FEW YEARS OF BEING MARRIED, RUNNING the studio, and working on my yoga-inspired rhymes, Amanda and I decided it was time to go back to India. We wanted to go back to Mysore to study with Pattabhi Jois, who was now in his late eighties. We also wanted to make a few pilgrimages. Amanda dreamt of visiting the fabled Ajanta caves, which were covered in two-thousand-year-old Buddhist murals. Years later, this experience would inspire Amanda on her own spiritual graffiti mission, to paint ten thousand Buddhas all over the world. I had a longing to visit Gandhi's ashram at Sevagram.

Gandhi was one of my heroes; his autobiography, *The Story of My Experiments with Truth,* was one of my favorite books. I loved reading about his transformation from a nervous and fearful young man into a great leader. As someone who grew up shy and who used to be terrified of public speaking, I found his story inspiring.

We arrived by train in the small town of Warda in the middle of the night. The station was littered with sleeping bodies, and we did our best to roll our luggage through the lobby without waking anyone up. Outside the station there was only one rickshaw. It was still dark when the driver dropped us off, and the gates to the ashram were locked. We sat down on the curb and waited; nowhere else to go.

An hour passed and a light rain began to fall. As dawn came and the sky turned a lighter shade of gray, large monkeys began talking and jumping around excitedly in the trees above us. At last a petite woman, wrapped in homespun khadi cloth, came and opened the gates. She welcomed us and brought us to a large, mostly vacant dormitory. Thin, dusty mattresses on iron cots lined the room. The place looked like it hadn't changed much since the 1930s. She invited us to get some rest and told us we could join in the lunchtime meal later that day.

When we woke up, we found our way to the kitchen area. Everyone who visits the ashram is asked to contribute with some daily chores. We learned how to sift rice over large, flat woven baskets so we could remove the pebbles before cooking.

A simple lunch of dhal and rice and some sautéed vegetables was served. Amanda looked over at me, wrinkling her nose. *What?* I mouthed. Then I took a bite. The food had no seasoning and no salt. After so many mouth-watering and delicious meals during my travels in India, this tasted like glue. I remember reading that Gandhi had been a strict vegetarian and believed that if one could conquer one's palette, one could conquer one's mind. He required that all salt, sugar, and spices be left out of his food so he could strengthen his willpower. It seemed like a strange practice, but as I stayed at the ashram and learned more about Gandhi's life, I realized that Gandhi had used his discipline to great advantage. He staged many long hunger strikes and through them had been able to turn the political tide and help to liberate India from the British. Gandhi taught that if you want to change the world you have to be willing to change yourself first.

In the mornings at the ashram, there was a prayer circle. It was an ecumenical service that included passages from all the different religious traditions. It was another way Gandhi reminded me to be open-minded, accepting, and inclusive. As days passed at the ashram, I began to appreciate the example that he had set, and a song about the life of Gandhi began to emerge. I decided to call it "Be the Change."

After a week at Sevagram we made our way to Mysore to practice again with Pattabhi Jois. Practicing yoga with Guruji was like receiving a vital transmission. The practice was strong, and left me feeling completely wrung out and deeply satisfied.

At the end of our two months in Mysore, I thought it would be fun to throw a free concert and share some of the new songs I had written. Anu's was a restaurant popular with the yogis; we ate there almost every day. When we shared our idea with the owner, Ganesh, he offered to host the event on the restaurant's rooftop. I met a German yogi, a percussionist who had just graduated from music school. He didn't have any drums with him, but he was still down to perform. Ingeniously, he created a drum kit for himself using a plastic shower bucket turned upside down and a couple of stainless-steel tiffin containers filled with rice as shakers. Ganesh was a tabla player and became the third member of our makeshift band. Amanda and I made a simple black-and-white flyer that read "YOGA HIP HOP FREE CONCERT," and wheat-pasted it around Mysore. To my amazement, word of mouth spread, and over a hundred people showed up.

We had no chairs, and everyone sat on the ground. Fortunately, it was a crowd of yogis, and no one seemed to mind. As we were about to start, we realized the rooftop was completely dark: there were no lights! Amanda MacGyvered two flashlights to create stage lighting.

For the next hour, with no sound system or microphone, I entertained our guests with hip-hop rhymes about Ganesh, Hanuman, Shiva, and yoga philosophy; Vedic verses about the chakras; and yoga science. The grand finale was my tribute to the life story of Mahatma Gandhi: the song "Be the Change" that I had written while visiting the ashram. The crowd went wild, and all participated in the call-and-response of the chorus. And so it was, on a rooftop in India, that MC YOGI was born.

WITH GREAT LOVE ANYTHING IS POSSIBLE

32

WITH GREAT LOVE ANYTHING IS POSSIBLE

NCOURAGED BY THE ENTHUSIASTIC RESPONSE from the yogis in India, I began the process of turning my yoga-inspired rhymes into songs. So far I'd written all my lyrics using beats from other people's music, and now I was ready to make my own. When I got home from India I began my search. That year I must have asked everyone I met if they or someone they knew could help me. "Do you make beats?" "Do you know *anyone* who makes beats?" It wasn't long until someone mentioned that Robin Livingston, a childhood friend, had a job as a sound engineer at a place called Conscious Sound Studios.

Conscious Sound was tucked in an old storage facility at the base of the Richmond Bridge, across the street from San Quentin penitentiary, the oldest prison in California. The recording studio was like a purple-and-blue psychedelic cave. The owner was a huge *Star Trek* fan, and the whole place felt like the starship *Enterprise.* Once Robin and I reconnected, we got right to work. I'd meet him after hours at the studio, after all his other sessions were finished, and he helped me create my first demos. I will always be so grateful to Robin. He believed in me from the start, when all I had was a bunch of notebooks filled with lyrics and an idea that I could make yoga-inspired hip-hop. We knocked out three tracks. The songs were raw, basic, and funky—old-school break beats against Indian samples and scratching. Those tracks became my first EP. When Robin asked me what I was going to call it, I thought about the letters *EP* and said, "Elephant Power!" It was my nod to Ganesh, the great elephant-headed deity, the remover of obstacles.

When we were done, Robin told me I really needed a producer—someone who could oversee the project—and also a budget. To make a whole album of finished songs would take an estimated $25,000 to $30,000 to cover studio time, session players, producer fees, mixing and mastering, etc. *Gulp.* My first major obstacle was now staring me in the face.

Amanda and I did not have that kind of money, not even close. At the time, I think that was our combined annual income for the studio. I figured I'd need a label to get this record made, but I had no idea how to go about finding one. I started to shop my demo around to anyone who would listen. Most people thought it was interesting and original but not commercially viable.

One record-industry veteran told me I needed to be angrier and have more angst, and that I should try to be more like Eminem.

One night, Amanda and I had dinner with some of the students from our yoga studio. As we sat around the table exchanging stories, someone asked me about my music project. I told our friends I didn't really know what to do, and that Robin and I were thinking about taking a road trip to Los Angeles to see if we could find anyone down there who might be interested in picking it up. That's when Steve, who ran the local bookstore with his wife, Kate, said to me, "You and Amanda have done so much for the community. Yoga has changed so many of our lives. I'm 100 percent positive that if you reached out for help on this project, you would discover you already have the support you need."

This idea was a revelation. That night after dinner, Amanda and I started to consider the idea of a fundraiser. We could offer a yoga class, a concert, and maybe some Indian food. It just might work, and it would be fun regardless. The next morning Steve and Kate came to class with a check for five hundred dollars. They wanted to be the first ones to support the record.

What happened after that blew my mind. Word started to spread, and even before we announced the fund-raiser, before anyone heard a single note of my music, people in the community, friends, and yoga students started to donate. People would literally just drive by our house and leave envelopes with checks and cash. Amanda's mom came to visit, and after she left we realized she had placed five hundred-dollar bills in between the branches of our houseplant, with a note saying she wanted to be one of the first to invest in MC YOGI. The night of the benefit, our yoga studio was packed to the rafters. Somehow we squeezed forty-four people into the room, which normally maxed out at thirty-five. It was mat on top of mat. And after the class, students poured into the barn, bodies steaming, to enjoy a night of music and, as promised, Indian food and chai. That night, we raised a remarkable thirteen thousand dollars. Another two thousand dollars flowed in the week after the event, and while we didn't have the total we needed, we had enough to get started. I had never thought that much about karma before. But that experience made me realize that the years of love and energy Amanda and I had poured into our community were now coming back to us tenfold.

So many amazing and talented people came together to help me create my first album. Sean Dinsmore, who pioneered hip-hop Indian fusion with the Dum Dum Project, flew in from Shanghai to produce. Three of the most famous *kirtan* singers in America—Krishna Das, Jai Uttal, and Bhagavan Das—all agreed to be guest singers on the album, and they all did it for free. Niraj Chag, a producer from London, contributed the music for the Gandhi track; Manose, a Nepalese rock star, lent his brilliant flute playing throughout; and Rita Sahai, known as the jewel of Indian music for her voice, sang as the goddess Parvati on the song "Son of Shiva."

Halfway through the project an independent label, White Swan Records, agreed to be our distributer and gave us the remaining funds we needed to finish the album as an advance.

One of the greatest blessings of making the album was getting to meet Sharon Gannon and David Life, the founders of Jivamukti yoga. Sean knew Sharon from his time in New York and had a feeling she would really appreciate the originality of the project. He made an introduction, and we asked her to sing on the song I had written about Krishna. Amanda and I fell in love with her and David right away; it was like an old soul connection. And they became two of our most influential teachers and friends.

When the album was finally finished, Sharon and David hosted the release party at their studio in New York City. The event marked the culmination of so many things—the end of my years of struggle as a teen, the creative pursuits of freestyling and graffiti art that were now focused in this unique way, all the years of practice as a yoga student, my trips to India, and the fulfillment of a desire I had so many years before to find a way to share my love of yoga with the world.

Through the unfolding of the entire process I felt that I had learned a deep lesson, something that Sharon taught me and something that I would always remember whenever I had a dream that seemed impossible. "With great love," Sharon would say, "anything is possible."

FESTIVALS STAGES AND PHASES

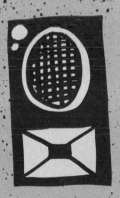

33

FESTIVALS, STAGES, AND PHASES

STOOD LIKE A DEER FROZEN IN THE HEADLIGHTS. I didn't know anything about anything. My album had come out and was starting to spread through the grassroots network of yoga teachers. I had just started to perform, and somehow through friends of friends I landed a performance slot on the main stage of major festival. The manager on the main stage was a grizzled veteran of the trade. As soon as I arrived to check in, he started barking at me: "You're late. I don't have an advance for you. Do you need a DI box? How many inputs???"

DI box? Inputs? My head swirled. I felt like I was going to throw up and then pass out. The reality of how completely inexperienced and unprepared I was hit me. Frustrated, the stage manager almost knocked me over as he rushed by, muttering under his breath, "Fucking amateurs."

When the invitation came in to perform, I called my friend Martin, aka Dragonfly, to DJ for me, and one of my oldest friends, Matty Love, agreed to back me up as a hype man. We never rehearsed together. I must have thought it would be easy, just freestyling and having fun like we did at the Shop.

I was feeling like a big shot, telling all my friends that I was performing on the main stage. It was the truth, but what I didn't know until I arrived on the festival grounds was that I was slated as a "tweener," or in-between act. I had a fifteen-minute slot that was meant to distract the audience while the crew struck the stage and set up for another main act. I was the tweener for the New Pornographers and a band called Kinky.

I looked over and heard the stage manager growling his commands at the rest of the crew, who moaned after every order. I stood backstage, in the shadows behind huge flight cases and crates, watching and observing as the stage crew struck the set, moving and hauling equipment. And then the moment of reckoning: "Get out there, kid." The stage manager waved me onstage.

I had fifteen minutes to show and prove. As I walked on it felt like I was walking the plank. Just as I took the stage the majority of the crowd turned and started walking away like a receding tide. Their favorite band had just finished, and now everyone was going to get a corn dog, nachos, and more beer. When Dragonfly dropped the beat, a few people stopped and turned around. There I was, knees shaking, voice cracking.

Matty grabbed the mic to hype the crowd, but there was no signal; his mic was dead. I looked at Martin for help. Martin held it down, but as I ran through my routine I realized we were in the dark. The lights were off and the stage was completely black. After about five minutes, Martin was able to wave down the light tech, and then, like a ray of sunshine breaking through the cloud cover, one single beam hit the stage. I stepped forward into the light. I looked over, and there was Matty, who was still in the dark. His mic was still off, but he was there; thank God he was there. Martin kept the groove going, and I did my best to perform my collection of yoga-inspired rhymes—which could easily have been the weirdest and most out-of-place thing at that entire festival.

I began a chorus and encouraged the audience to clap along with me. I could see some hands clapping, some heads beginning to nod. *This is working*, I thought to myself, *it's actually working!* Then, as I was starting to hit my stride and my confidence was growing, I heard a thunderous sound coming from behind me onstage. *CRACK!* The intense sound cut through the mix like an axe chopping through the hull of a ship. And then again, *BOOM CRACK! BOOM BOOM CRACK!* The offbeat sound started to throw me off my rhythm. I turned around, and that's when I saw the sound technician, hunched over, smoking a cigarette, looking like he'd just woken up from a drunken nap. He was checking the drums for the next band. I looked at him pleadingly as if to say, *Hey, man, I am actually trying to perform right now.* He just continued to bang away on the drums with an expression on his face that I read as *Screw you and your hippie friends.*

Everything that could go wrong, went wrong. My ship sunk that night; I felt worthless. At the end of our pathetic set, Matty pumped his fist in the air like the true friend and champion that he is. I dropped the mic, and not in the cool, "I just destroyed the crowd" kind of way, but in a completely ruined, soul-crushed, "I never want to do this again" kind of way.

I felt completely humiliated. As the music finished, a cluster of claps and very light applause followed, but I couldn't hear it. The host came out, and instead of acknowledging our little tweener act, he pumped the crowd for the next band.

Amanda met me backstage with a huge hug, like a blanket of love. I couldn't wait to get as far away from that stage as possible. We wandered through the dust-covered fields of the festival together. It was night, and most of the eyes of the crowd were blood-red, like zombies. The massive crowd of festival punks, drunks, and freaks ebbed and flowed, drifting in and out in search of the next attraction, the next high.

We wandered toward the electronic dome, where a friend was deejaying. As we meandered down the path, I felt my entire spirit sag. *Maybe this music thing isn't meant to be,* I thought.

Then something caught my attention; there was an energy in front of me. I lifted my eyes, and there like a lighthouse stood a massive statue of Shiva. The huge brass god stood in a dancing pose. The statue was wrapped in Christmas lights, with heaps of flowers all around him. *Maybe this is a sign,* I thought. Shiva is the god of destruction, and I'd just had my ego obliterated onstage.

During my time in India I learned that the devastation caused by Shiva is only to make way for new creation. It serves a divine purpose. Shiva destroys our ignorance, our fears, our arrogance, so we can rise up and dance again. I realized then that I had just received a brutal but necessary lesson. It was a rite of passage into the world of being a professional performer. In that moment, I saw the perfection of everything that had just happened and knew that my only option was to keep going, to pick myself back up and try again.

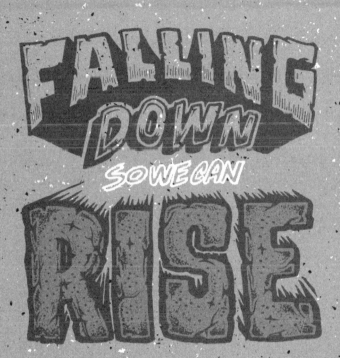

34

FALLING DOWN
SO WE CAN RISE

IDIDN'T GIVE UP. I WAS BECOMING MORE RESILIENT, and the discipline of my yoga practice was helping me to cope with the ups and downs of being a performer. The next stage was smaller, but the reception was much bigger. When I looked out at the audience I saw kids who knew my lyrics, which was an amazing feeling. I started getting phone calls and messages from people inviting me to festivals and events all across the country, my first album was charting on iTunes, and the momentum was building. Around the time when things were really starting to pick up, I got a terrible phone call. My teacher Larry was in the hospital in a coma.

We held vigil all week, chanting and praying for him. Amanda and I were on tour in Texas when it became clear that he was not going to come out of his coma. His wife and longtime students were by his side in the hospital. We called, and they held the phone up to his ear. I whispered my gratitude to my teacher as tears streamed down my face. "You saved my life, Larry. You took me under your wing, you introduced me to Amanda, you helped me find my purpose, and my path. *Om Namah Shivaya,*" I chanted softly. "May God welcome you home with open arms. *Om Namah Shivaya.*" As my voice trailed off, I handed the phone to Amanda so she could say her good-byes.

When we finished the call, we realized we had been parked outside the Rothko Chapel in Houston. We wiped the tears from our faces and went in. The chapel was in a modern, minimalist octagonal building. Inside, fourteen large paintings in black hues by the artist Mark Rothko graced the walls. We sat in silence on the bench inside, gazing into the darkness of the paintings. At first the large black canvases looked empty, but after some time I started to see all the subtle variations. What looked at first like emptiness, like death, was actually scintillating energy, pure potentiality, life. Sacred books lined a thin shelf along one of the walls—copies of the Bible, the Koran, the Bhagavad Gita, *A Course in Miracles.* We sifted through them for some guidance, some inspiration, and then offered our own prayers silently into the space: *May Larry's passing be peaceful. May he know how much he is loved.* A brochure told us that the purpose of the chapel was "to inspire people to action through art and contemplation and to nurture reverence for the highest aspirations of humanity."

A few hours later, we received the news: Larry had left his body. That night I saw one of the biggest and brightest shooting stars I'd ever seen in my life. The Rocket Man was gone, but behind him he left a trail of light, and a legacy of love.

A group of Larry's friends, family, and students held a memorial service for him in the streets of SOMA. We lit candles and shared stories. That night when I got home I received an email. It was an invitation to headline a huge festival.

I'd opened for other headliners before, from Ziggy Marley and Moby to Michael Franti and Matisyahu, but I'd never been one of the main acts at an event of that size. I told Amanda about the offer, and she told me to go for it. I made a few calls, we booked our flights, and the next thing you know I was backstage at the festival, looking out across a sea of ten thousand people. The promoter said there would be over twenty thousand people throughout the day. My stomach tightened.

I stood nervously backstage, getting ready for my set. There was a thin layer of dust being picked up by the wind; I covered my face to shield my eyes. As I looked up I could see my friend DJ Drez setting up his turntables, making sure everything was plugged in and the needles were ready.

As the host announced my name, I ran my fingers nervously against my prayer beads, chanting to myself to calm my nerves and gather my courage. Feeling the beads under my fingers, I was flooded with memories of everything that led me to this point. I remembered how Prakash had taught me how to chant using the beads . . . I flashed back to my time in India, learning from Acharya that things take time and are a process . . . I remembered seeing Amanda for the first time . . . practicing with Larry every day . . . the first time I did yoga with my dad . . . the way that finding yoga steered me away from a dangerous path onto a better one . . . I thought of my teachers and all the people who had helped me along the way. As I made the long, slow walk to the front of the stage, I looked out across the sea of human beings. The crowd swelled as people moved in and out; it was like looking at one massive living organism. Bright rays from the sun poured in over the hills, flooding the field that stretched out in front of me. The warm glare of gold crossed my face and made me squint. I took a deep breath, and felt the oxygen spreading across my lungs. I reached for the mic and clutched it with my sweaty palm. I could feel my pulse throbbing in my hand as I gripped the metal microphone.

Security flanked both sides like royal guards, making sure no one climbed onto the stage. I looked across the platform at Drez to see if he was ready to drop the first beat. He nodded and let me know we were good to go.

I heard Larry's voice in my head: "You're stronger than you think you are, Lucky. You've got this." I was suddenly flooded with a huge wave of energy. All my doubts vanished, and instinctively I raised my right arm in the sky, extending my pointer finger to the sun. One arm in the front row followed suit; then the whole front section caught the wave, ten arms turned into twenty, twenty became a hundred. Within seconds I looked out and saw ten thousand arms raised to the sky. It felt like we were all one. With great gusto I let my voice break through the speakers: "Check, check . . . WHO'S READY TO RISE UP!?!"

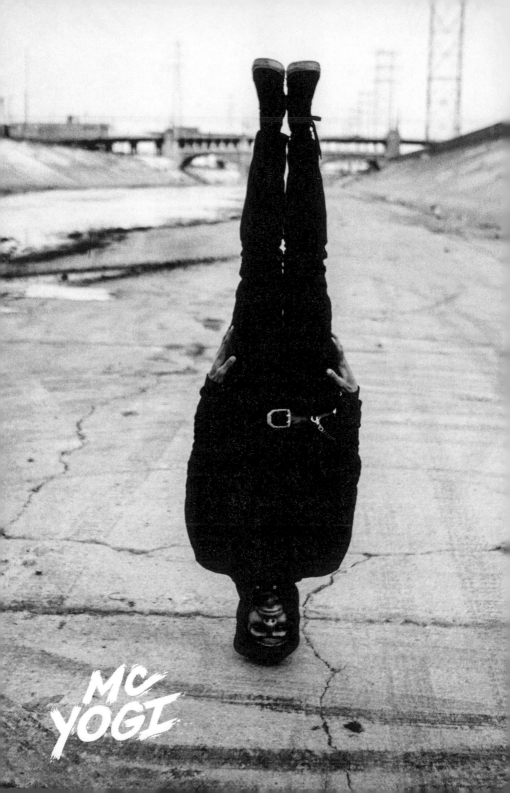

ACKNOWLEDGMENTS

I'M BLESSED TO HAVE ONE OF THE BEST FAMILIES, WHO have loved and supported me through all the phases and stages of my life, starting with my wife, Amanda; my mom and dad; my sister, Melissa; and my brother, Adam. Tina, David, and Sam B.; Nancy Merrill, John and Carol Merrill.

To my teachers and mentors, thank you for all your wisdom and guidance; without you I would still be lost, wandering in the dark: Larry Schultz, Dorothy Divack, Gurumayi Chidvilasananda, Shri K. Pattabhi Jois and his family, Yogacharya Venkatesh and Hemalaya, Sharon Gannon, David Life, Tim Miller, Chuck Miller, Shiva Rea, Rod Stryker, Peggy Orr, the monks at the Vedanta Society in Olema, California, and all the students, teachers, and friends at Point Reyes Yoga.

To my editor, Katy Hamilton, and the whole team at HarperOne, thank you for your kindness, patience, and support, and for giving me this opportunity to tell my story.

Thank you to Estevan Oriol for your incredible eye and artistic talent in creating the photos we used for this book.

To my N3W LEVEL family: This book would not have happened without the visionary instincts of Tim Cook and the support of the whole N3W LEVEL squad, including Isabelle Abergel and Rachel White. I'm so grateful for your support.

To all my friends and colleagues who have supported my journey: John Crews for giving me a second chance; my friends and the staff at the group home; Vivek, Surendar, and Ram, White Swan Records, Parmita Pushman and Joel Davis for believing in me from the start; B2 in Hong Kong, Jonathon Serbin, and Sean Dinsmore; Clive and Eriko, Bharat Mitra, Noah Levine and the Dharma Punx crew; Leza Lowitz, for your invaluable feedback on an early draft; the Wanderlust crew—Jeff Krasno and Schuyler Grant, Sean and Karina Hoess; my awesome assistant Melissa McLaughlin, for your daily support and friendship.

And to my extended yoga and music fam: DJ Drez and Marti Nikko, Robin Livingston, Mike Green, East Forest, Sianna Sherman, Janet Stone, Elena Brower, Chris Cuevos and Anne Marie Kramer, Krishna Das, Jai Uttal, and Bhagavan Das; Trevor and Emory Hall, DJ Dragonfly, Sol Rising, Katie Cariffe, Yoga Robb, Rachel and Duke, Matthew and Avasa Love, Steve Costa and Kate Levinson, Kel, Basta, Emil, Jomial, Swannie. And lastly you, for sharing this journey.

Peace and love,
MC YOGI

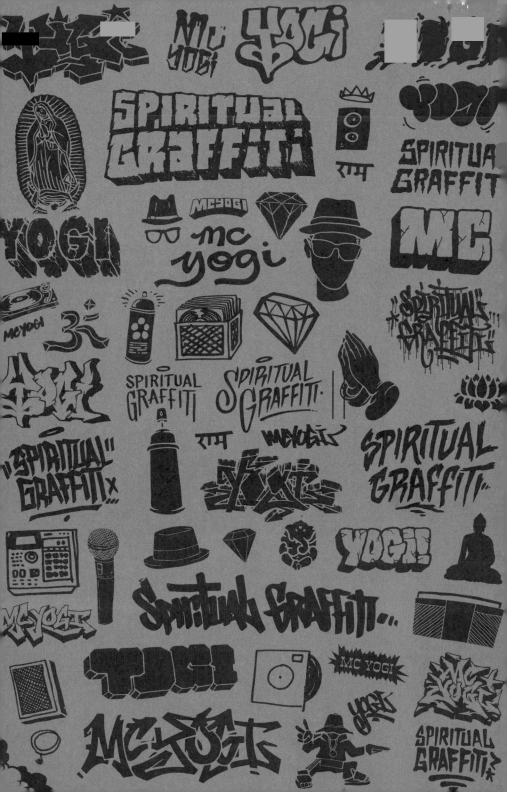